Understanding
Stroke

Professor Richard Iain Lindley

Published by Family Doctor Publications Limited
in association with the British Medical Association

IMPORTANT

This book is intended not as a substitute for personal medical advice but as a supplement to that advice for the patient who wishes to understand more about his or her condition.

Before taking any form of treatment
YOU SHOULD ALWAYS CONSULT YOUR MEDICAL PRACTITIONER.

In particular (without limit) you should note that advances in medical science occur rapidly and some information about drugs and treatment contained in this booklet may very soon be out of date.

Acknowledgements
The following people read early drafts of this book and the author is grateful for their helpful suggestions and comments: Campbell Chalmers, Martin Dennis, John and Mary Lindley, Lesley Moffat and Mark Smith; Joan Brodie provided additional information. Paul O'Mahony provided valuable advice for the recent revision. I'd like to thank the Western General Hospital, Westmead Hospital and Blacktown Hospital Stroke Teams for their support and advice and my patients for teaching me the things that really matter.

Family Doctor Publications, PO Box 4664, Poole, Dorset BH15 1NN

ISBN-13: 978-1-903474-99-0
ISBN-10: 1-903474-99-X

20002011

Contents

Patient experiences

Sharing knowledge and experience of ill health

Many people who have experienced ill health are much wiser as a result.

On our website (www.familydoctor.co.uk) we are creating a resource where people who wish to know more about an illness or condition can learn from other people's experiences of that illness.

If you have had a health experience that may be useful to someone in a similar situation, we invite you to share this by clicking on the 'Patient Experience' tab at www.familydoctor.co.uk (see below).

- Your 'Patient Experience' will be completely anonymous – there will be no link back to you and we require no personal information from you.

- Your 'Patient Experience' will not be a forum or discussion – there is no opportunity for others to comment either positively or negatively on what you have written.

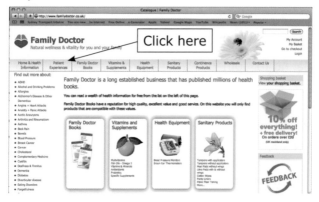

About the author

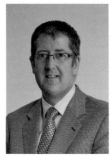

Richard Lindley is the Moran Foundation for Older Australians Professor of Geriatric Medicine at the University of Sydney. He has had a special interest in stroke medicine for over 20 years and completed his research doctorate with the Edinburgh Stroke Group. He has participated in many of the clinical trials that have improved the care for people with stroke, and is currently running trials of acute thrombolysis treatment for ischaemic stroke, blood pressure lowering for haemorrhagic stroke, and early and intense mobilisation rehabilitation after stroke. He remains a stroke clinician at Blacktown Hospital in Sydney. In 2010 he was elected the President of the Stroke Society of Australasia.

Introduction

This book is about strokes. A stroke occurs when part of the brain is damaged as a result of a lack of blood supply or the rupture of a blood vessel – a haemorrhage. Some strokes cause catastrophic collapse with a sudden loss of consciousness. These types of stroke are usually caused by a massive brain haemorrhage, and are so characteristic that the ancient Greeks coined the term 'apoplexy', an old name for a stroke. Another old term for a stroke is 'cerebrovascular accident'. A stroke is certainly not an accident and is often the result of decades of wear and tear and 'furring up' of the blood vessels supplying the brain. However, the abbreviation 'CVA' (for cerebrovascular accident) is still commonly used.

In the United Kingdom, over 110,000 people have a stroke for the first time each year. This is a rate of around 2 per 1,000 people annually. The risk of a stroke increases with age and is higher in men than in women.

Strokes are so common that most of us will know a friend or a relative who has had one. Until fairly recently, however, stroke has not been a major medical priority, perhaps because many of the people having one were old or simply too disabled to make much fuss. But stroke should not be ignored. It is the third most common cause of death in the UK and one of the major causes of serious disability. During the 1990s, health services for stroke and stroke research were made a government priority, but by the end of the twentieth century stroke seemed to have slipped down the priority list (dominated by heart disease, cancer and mental health). However, the last decade has seen an explosion of interest in stroke services and research. Doctors are now wiser and recognise that much can be done to prevent a stroke, treat, and sometimes reverse, the stroke itself and improve the outcome through an organised rehabilitation programme.

Many people confuse a stroke with a heart attack. There are similarities, in that heart attacks are caused by blood vessels becoming blocked in the heart and strokes result from blood supply problems in the brain. However, heart attacks tend to occur with sudden chest and arm pain (together with faintness, panic and sickness), whereas strokes are usually painless and occur with various combinations of symptoms including a sudden loss of movement and problems with speech, vision and/or balance.

Recently, a group of stroke experts suggested changing the name of stroke to 'brain attack' to raise awareness among both the medical profession and the public that the brain is just as important as the heart.

KEY POINTS

- Strokes are very common and are one of the major causes of death and disability in the UK

- After years of neglect, stroke is now getting a high priority

- Strokes affect the brain and are usually painless

- A stroke is not the same as a heart attack

- Heart attacks usually start with a sudden tightness or pain in the chest

What is a stroke?

The brain controls our body movements, processes information from the outside world and allows us to communicate with others. A stroke occurs when part of the brain stops working because of problems with its blood supply. This leads to the classic symptoms of a stroke, such as a sudden weakness affecting the arm and leg on the same side of the body.

The brain is one of the most delicate parts of the body and, tragically, even a short time without a good blood supply can be disastrous. For example, although a finger or even a leg can be successfully saved after many hours without a blood supply, the brain is damaged within minutes. The symptoms of a stroke usually come on quickly and can be very severe.

Brain function

It is useful to describe the structure of the brain to help understand why different sorts of strokes occur.

The brain is encased in the bony skull and communicates with the rest of the body through the cranial nerves (which pass through openings in the

Nerve network

The brain controls body movement, processes information from the outside world and allows us to communicate with others through a network of nerves that range throughout the body.

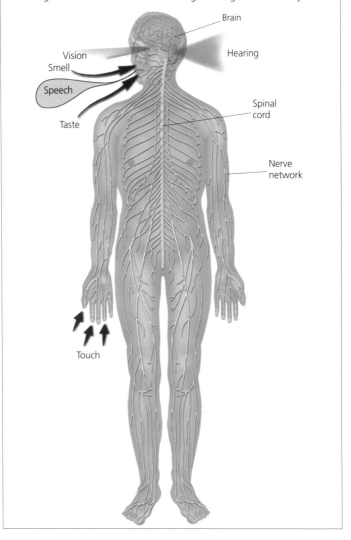

Structure of the brain

The brain has two hemispheres: the left and the right. Each hemisphere is composed of four lobes. Each of the four lobes of each cerebral hemisphere has its own particular physical and mental functions. These can be impaired by brain damage.

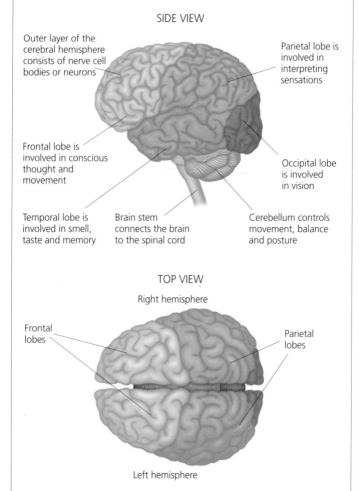

SIDE VIEW

Outer layer of the cerebral hemisphere consists of nerve cell bodies or neurons

Parietal lobe is involved in interpreting sensations

Frontal lobe is involved in conscious thought and movement

Occipital lobe is involved in vision

Temporal lobe is involved in smell, taste and memory

Brain stem connects the brain to the spinal cord

Cerebellum controls movement, balance and posture

TOP VIEW

Right hemisphere

Frontal lobes

Parietal lobes

Left hemisphere

skull) and the spinal nerves (which pass from the spinal cord through small gaps between the bones of the spine and control the arms, trunk and legs). The brain is made up of three main regions:

1 the brain stem
2 the cerebellum
3 the cerebral hemispheres.

The brain stem controls the breathing, heart rate and important reflexes, for example, the cough reflex to clear the breathing tubes. The 'cerebellum' is the centre for balance and coordination of movement. In evolutionary terms; these parts of the brain are quite old and provide the minimum brain power to survive. Connected to this more primitive part of the brain are the two cerebral hemispheres (left and right), which control speech, thinking, complex movements and vision.

The right and left hemispheres communicate through nerve fibre bundles that cross from one side of the body to the other. As a result, the left side of the brain controls the right side of the body and vice versa. A stroke affecting the left side of the brain therefore causes symptoms (for example, weakness) in the right side of the body. In most right-handed people, the left hemisphere is dominant and controls logic and speech, whereas the right hemisphere is involved with imagination and creative thought. This is called left-sided dominance.

The blood supply to the brain is from four main blood vessels – two vertebral arteries and two carotid arteries. The vertebral arteries enter the skull from the backbone and mainly supply the brain stem and

Crossover

The right and left hemispheres communicate with the muscles and sense organs through nerve bundles that cross from one side of the brain to the other. As a result, the left side of the brain controls the right side of the body and vice versa.

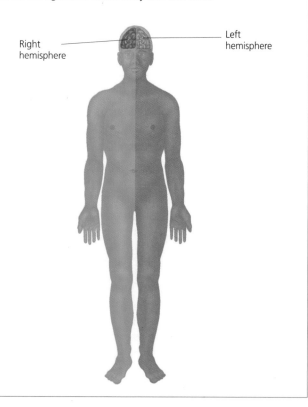

Right
hemisphere

Left
hemisphere

cerebellum, whereas the two carotid arteries enter the skull from the front of the neck and mainly supply the two cerebral hemispheres.

All four arteries join up in a rough circle, which helps to maintain an adequate supply of blood if one artery gets blocked. Water mains and electricity

Brain arteries

The blood is supplied to the brain from the front of the neck and the backbone. The arteries join in a rough circle which helps to maintain an adequate supply of blood if one artery is blocked.

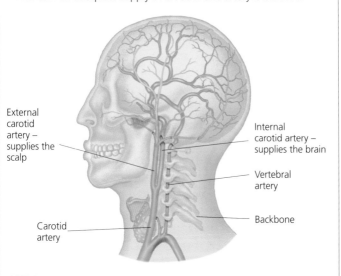

External carotid artery – supplies the scalp

Internal carotid artery – supplies the brain

Vertebral artery

Backbone

Carotid artery

supplies operate on similar principles, to try to maintain adequate supplies even if part of the supply breaks down. Unfortunately, the effectiveness of the circle of arteries varies from person to person and often does not protect people from the symptoms of a stroke if one of the main arteries becomes blocked.

Causes of a stroke

The brain uses large amounts of oxygen and nutrients (for example, glucose), which are supplied through the circulation. The most common cause of a stroke is when a blood vessel supplying these vital nutrients to the brain becomes blocked with a blood clot. The blood clot – known as a thrombosis – may form locally in a brain artery or form elsewhere (for example, in the heart) and travel in the bloodstream to lodge in the brain.

This type of wandering clot is known as an embolus. When a blood vessel in the brain becomes blocked, the brain cells that it supplies quickly become starved of oxygen and glucose, and stop working properly. If the blood supply is not quickly resumed, these brain cells will die. This type of stroke is called an ischaemic stroke, or a 'cerebral infarct'. The medical term 'ischaemic' means a shortage of blood. 'Cerebral' is the medical term for the brain and 'infarct' is the medical term for death of a part of the body.

The second most common cause of a stroke is a brain haemorrhage, which occurs when a blood vessel bursts inside the head. As well as disrupting the supply

Thrombosis

The most common cause of a stroke is a thrombosis – when a blood vessel supplying vital nutrients to the brain becomes blocked with a blood clot.

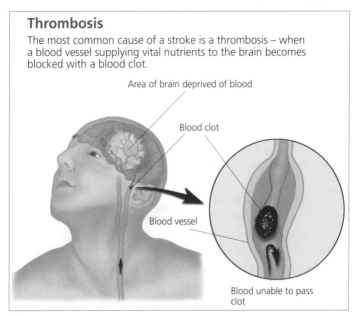

Area of brain deprived of blood

Blood clot

Blood vessel

Blood unable to pass clot

Brain bleed

The second most common cause of a stroke is a brain haemorrhage, which occurs when a blood vessel bursts inside the head.

Skin

Skull bone

Dura mater

Subarachnoid space

Pia mater

Arachnoid

Subarachnoid haemorrhage – blood escapes and fills subarachnoid space

Intracerebral haemorrhage – blood collects within the brain

of oxygen and glucose to some parts of the brain, the escaping blood can cause damage by clotting, swelling and triggering inflammation.

There are two types of brain haemorrhage: an intracerebral haemorrhage, when blood collects within the brain, and a subarachnoid haemorrhage, when blood collects between the skull and the brain.

Doctors are now recognising some medical conditions that appear to weaken blood vessels and increase the chance of a rupture. High blood pressure certainly seems to be an important cause of an intracerebral haemorrhage. Subarachnoid haemorrhage is mainly caused by the rupture of small swellings – known as aneurysms – which can form in weakened blood vessels, and this problem can run in families.

Any bleed or thromboembolus within the head that causes a loss of function for more than 24 hours (assuming that the patient survives) can be called a stroke. Symptoms that last less than 24 hours, and from which there is a complete recovery, are known as a transient ischaemic attack (TIA) or mini-stroke (see 'Types of strokes', page 14). There is now an increased tendency to call any attack that leads to changes on a brain scan a 'stroke', leaving the term 'TIA' for events that last less than 24 hours and leave no evidence of damage on the brain scan. These new definitions are likely to become more widely used over the next few years.

It is often difficult to tell an ischaemic cerebral stroke from a haemorrhagic stroke. Both can cause weakness, numbness or paralysis of part of the body, and may be associated with slurred speech and a loss of consciousness. A haemorrhagic stroke is often accompanied by a severe headache, however, and can be more severe, with widespread damage, so that a prolonged loss of consciousness (coma) is more likely. Only a brain scan can reliably determine what type of stroke has occurred (haemorrhage or ischaemia).

KEY POINTS

- Strokes result from problems affecting the blood supply to the brain

- Some strokes are caused by the blockage of a blood vessel with a blood clot

- Some strokes occur when a blood vessel ruptures

Types of strokes

The symptoms of a stroke depend on which part of the brain has been damaged. Any part of the blood vessel system can become blocked so there are many varieties of stroke. The blood supply to the brain also varies a surprising amount from person to person. Some people can block three of their four main arteries and not have a stroke. Others may have a devastating stroke with a blockage of just one of the four arteries. This has led to great difficulty in classifying strokes and there are many different classifications in use around the world.

A stroke on the left side of the brain

A stroke affecting the right side of the body is usually the result of problems in the left side of the brain (and vice versa). For more details on the functions of the left and right side of the brain, see 'What is a stroke?' (page 4).

The most familiar type of stroke is when someone suddenly develops a weakness of the right (or left) side of the face, arm and leg. This problem is easy to spot, and the medical term is a 'hemiparesis' or

Writing

A stroke affecting the right side of the body is usually the result of problems in the left side of the brain.

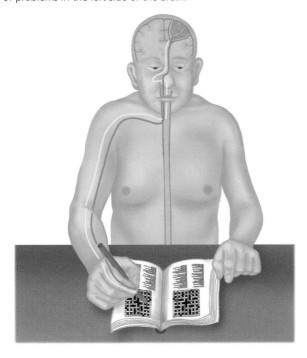

a 'hemiplegia' (commonly shortened to 'hemi'). The weakness can vary from very mild to complete paralysis. It most often affects the face, arm and leg together, but some small strokes just affect the face alone or just the arm or the leg. Less commonly, strokes can cause just a loss of feeling (or sensation) in the face, arm or leg, or a mixture of a loss of feeling and weakness.

Although weakness is the obvious initial symptom of a stroke, the increased stiffness that develops later can cause many other problems. This stiffness is called spasticity and occurs in muscles that have lost their nerve supply and are not used regularly. If people do not get good rehabilitation after their stroke, the spasticity can lead to painful spasms and abnormal posture. Physiotherapy aims to restore normal movements and the early sessions often concentrate on reducing any spasticity of the affected arm and leg.

If your only problem after a stroke is a weakness down one side of your body, this suggests that the stroke has been slight and damaged only a small area of 'wiring' deep in your brain. If, however, the stroke has damaged a much larger area of your brain, other things are affected too.

Cortex functions

Different areas of the cortex have specific functions. The symptoms of a stroke depend on which part of the brain has been damaged.

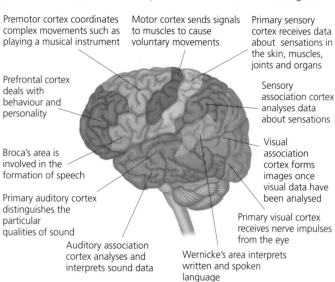

Premotor cortex coordinates complex movements such as playing a musical instrument

Motor cortex sends signals to muscles to cause voluntary movements

Primary sensory cortex receives data about sensations in the skin, muscles, joints and organs

Prefrontal cortex deals with behaviour and personality

Sensory association cortex analyses data about sensations

Broca's area is involved in the formation of speech

Visual association cortex forms images once visual data have been analysed

Primary auditory cortex distinguishes the particular qualities of sound

Primary visual cortex receives nerve impulses from the eye

Auditory association cortex analyses and interprets sound data

Wernicke's area interprets written and spoken language

In right-handed people, the left side of the brain usually controls language, an ability to see the world on the right, and an ability to recognise and coordinate things on the right. Therefore, larger strokes affecting the left side of the brain can cause a more severe combination of right-sided weakness, an inability to speak and an inability to see objects to the right. In left-handed people, these functions are usually controlled by the right side of the brain, although this is not an absolute rule.

Case history

A retired managing director suddenly collapsed while standing in the kitchen. He fell onto the tiled floor and bruised himself badly. He didn't lose consciousness and managed to shout for help. When seen at the stroke unit, his mouth had drooped down on the right and he couldn't move his right arm or leg at all. His speech was normal and he could feel normal sensations down the right side of his body.

A brain scan using a technique called computed tomography (CT) showed a small area of damage deep in the left side of his brain, consistent with a blockage affecting a small blood vessel. His weakness rapidly improved and, after four weeks of rehabilitation at the stroke unit, he went home almost independent and able to climb stairs.

Problems affecting speech

Speech problems that occur with a stroke commonly involve a difficulty in mentally formulating and understanding the right words to use. People who recover from the language problem tell of the frustration that it causes. Patients say that they knew

Mind map

Each side of the brain has its own sensory and motor cortices which sense touch and control movement in the opposite side of the body. Movements that involve great complexity or parts of the body that are very sensitive to touch are allocated proportionally larger areas of processing cortex.

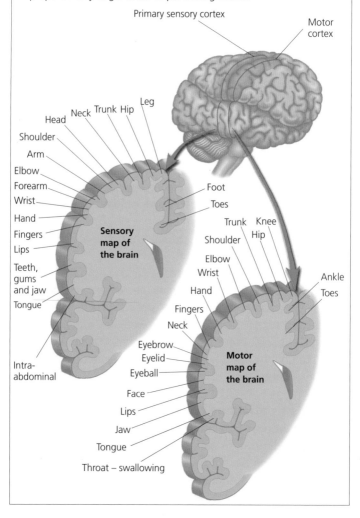

Primary sensory cortex

Motor cortex

Head
Neck Trunk Hip
Leg
Shoulder
Arm
Elbow
Forearm
Wrist
Hand
Fingers
Lips
Teeth, gums and jaw
Tongue

Sensory map of the brain

Foot
Toes

Intra-abdominal

Trunk Knee
Shoulder Hip
Elbow
Wrist
Hand
Fingers
Neck
Eyebrow
Eyelid
Eyeball

Motor map of the brain

Ankle
Toes

Face
Lips
Jaw
Tongue
Throat – swallowing

what to say but were unable to get the words out in the right order. This can be very mild, such as an inability to recall the name of a common object such as a watch, or more severe and mean a complete loss of all speech. This problem is called aphasia or dysphasia.

Sometimes, a different type of speech problem occurs as a result of weakness of the muscles involved in moving the mouth and tongue when articulating words – this is known as dysarthria.

Which side of your brain is dominant?

- Most people who are right-handed will be left brain dominant and strokes affecting the left side of their brain can cause language problems (dysphasia)
- About 50% of people who are naturally left-handed will also have left brain dominance and strokes affecting the left side of their brain can also cause language problems
- About 50% of people who are naturally left-handed will have right brain dominance, and strokes affecting the right side of their brain can cause language problems
- Many older people who were naturally left-handed were forced to use their non-dominant hand to write, and so appear right-handed. Half of these patients will have right brain dominance
- Doctors will try to assess dominance by asking you whether you are right- or left-handed AND by asking you which hand you prefer to use when picking up objects

Case history

A retired teacher aged 70 was talking to her daughter on the telephone. Her daughter reported that her mother's speech suddenly changed to 'gibberish' yet her mother was unaware of the problem. Mrs Smith had just had a stroke affecting the part of the brain that controls the production of speech. This symptom is called dysphasia.

A stroke on the right side of the brain

The left side of the body is controlled by the right side of the brain and in right-handed people this is normally the non-dominant side. The problems are very similar to the 'right-sided' problems described above, but language problems are much less common.

One common problem seen in people with larger strokes affecting the left side of the body is that they often appear very disabled and it is difficult to see why at first. This problem is the result of a failure of the brain to recognise that the left arm and leg actually belong to that person. The part of the brain that tells you that you have a left arm and leg is so damaged that your brain assumes that you don't have a left-hand side. When this is really severe, people can even ignore food on the left side of their plate, and 'lose' their left arm and leg.

Another pattern recognised in people with a left-sided weakness is abnormal speech, when the speech becomes rather monotonous or flat. The sing-song nature of speech that makes conversation more interesting and animated seems to be controlled by the right (or non-dominant) side of the brain.

Left-handedness

If you are naturally left-handed, the dominant side of your brain could be on the right or the left. Left-handed people may have a slightly different combination of stroke symptoms to those described above.

Problems affecting vision

The most common problem affecting eyesight is an inability to see the world on the right (or the left) as a result of problems in the brain on the left (or the right). This is because vision from the left field (side) of both eyes is controlled by the right side of the brain and vice versa.

This loss of a visual field is often mistaken for blindness in an eye, but in fact it involves a loss of vision in one field of both eyes. This type of visual field loss is called a hemianopia. However, most strokes do not damage the eye, but affect the processing of information from the eye. Double vision can also be caused by a stroke if the balance and coordination centre of the brain is affected, although many other non-stroke conditions can also cause double vision.

Problems affecting balance

The base of the brain has a complicated set of 'wiring' and control mechanisms to stop you falling over. Strokes affecting this area of the brain can cause sudden unsteadiness, and many patients say the problem is just like being drunk.

Transient ischaemic attacks

Some stroke symptoms disappear very quickly and within minutes (or hours) you are back to normal. If the stroke symptoms last less than 24 hours, doctors call the attack a transient ischaemic attack (TIA), a sort of mini-stroke. If the symptoms last more than 24 hours, the name 'stroke' is preferred. A TIA may be caused by a small blood clot that quickly breaks up, or a temporarily reduced blood flow in the brain (for example, as a result of an abnormal heart rhythm, low blood pressure or spasm of narrowed blood vessels).

A special form of a TIA affects the vision in one eye. This is called amaurosis fugax, or transient monocular blindness. A typical attack is when the vision in one eye disappears as if a black shutter was coming up or down. The attacks are sometimes described as a sudden misting of vision. You can test whether the problem is in both eyes or just the one eye by covering each eye in turn.

If your loss of vision is affecting just one eye and your vision recovers in seconds or minutes, this is usually the result of circulation problems affecting the blood supply to your eye (which is shared by your brain). The blood clot usually comes from a particular source, such as damage or disease affecting the heart or the carotid arteries (the blood vessels supplying blood to the head). These sorts of attacks can also be a warning of a future stroke, because the next time the blood clot may go to the brain, and not the eye. Early medical treatment can prevent the potential future major stroke after such an eye attack so this should be treated as a medical emergency.

A TIA is not a trivial attack and is a warning that there may be problems with the circulation. People who have had a TIA have a greater than normal risk of another attack which may be more serious, for example, a disabling stroke. It is therefore important that any stroke-like attack should be assessed by your doctor, who may be able to suggest ways of preventing more serious attacks in the near future.

Case history

A 65-year-old woman was smoking a cigarette when she suddenly dropped it. When she tried to pick it up, she found that her right hand was weak and she couldn't grip her fingers tight enough. When she tried to get up out of the chair, she noticed that her right leg wasn't moving. She waited five minutes and tried again, and managed to get to the telephone and call her son. When the son arrived 30 minutes later, she had regained full power in her hand and leg and felt back to normal. She had experienced a TIA, which can be an early warning of a more serious stroke yet to come.

Conditions that mimic a stroke

Many conditions can mimic a stroke, including the following.

Brain tumours

The main characteristic of a stroke is that the symptoms come on very quickly. A brain tumour can cause exactly the same problems as a stroke, but the symptoms tend to start gradually and get worse over days and weeks. Stroke-like symptoms that get worse need urgent medical attention from your doctor.

Migraine

Migraine is a very common condition, and some people experience a variety of symptoms with their attacks, with flashing lights, holes in their vision and even occasional arm or leg weakness. This can sometimes be difficult to treat and control, and some migraine attacks can be mistaken for a stroke. To complicate matters further, on rare occasions a migraine attack can lead to a stroke. An expert medical opinion may help in this situation.

Pins and needles

The sensation of pins and needles is a very common symptom and is only rarely caused by a stroke. More commonly, these symptoms are the result of a trapped nerve and have nothing to do with a stroke.

Eye symptoms

Symptoms such as a temporary loss of vision, blurred vision or double vision could result from a stroke, but are also signs of other serious problems affecting the eye. These symptoms should be assessed urgently by your family doctor. 'Floaters', small moving shapes that sometimes move across your vision, are not the result of a stroke and are usually normal.

Fits (or seizures)

These can occasionally mimic a stroke. Major fits often start with a collapse, and the person is unresponsive. The person's arms and legs jerk in a rhythmical manner for a few minutes, followed by a quieter recovery period. The fit may cause incontinence of urine or faeces, and sometimes people find that they have bitten their tongue. Some people have a weakness just like a stroke immediately after a fit and, if the doctor wasn't aware of the full attack, they may mistakenly diagnose a stroke. A witness can be very important to tell the two events apart, especially if a typical epileptic fit is seen.

KEY POINTS

- A stroke is characterised by a sudden onset of symptoms that can cause a wide range of different problems

- Strokes commonly cause arm and leg paralysis, speech problems, visual problems and coordination difficulties

- Minor stroke-like attacks, which completely resolve within a day, are called transient ischaemic attacks, or TIAs

- TIAs carry an increased risk of future strokes and therefore must be taken seriously

- Many conditions can mimic a stroke, including brain tumours, epileptic fits and migraine attacks

Why have you had a stroke?

It is surprisingly difficult to tell why someone has just had a stroke. Although a great deal is known about the causes of a stroke, the evidence often disappears in the initial stages. For example, if the stroke was caused by a blood clot that has travelled from an abnormality in the heart, a heart scan – carried out to try to find the source of a suspected embolus – will often fail to provide evidence of an abnormal blood clot. This is because the offending clot is now in the brain, having caused the stroke.

Strokes can affect the very young (even tiny children), but are very rare at this age. As our population ages, the average age of a person with a stroke is about 75 years. Stroke gets more common with increasing age; however, better stroke prevention has reduced the general risk of stroke.

These two factors have worked in opposite directions (ageing society increasing the number of strokes and better prevention decreasing the number), and overall the numbers of people having strokes in the UK have remained fairly constant over the past two decades. The chance of an 80 year old having a stroke is about 30 times greater than the chance of a 50 year old having one. This is probably the result of wear and tear of the blood vessels, accelerated by high blood pressure, smoking, diabetes and high cholesterol. Not a lot can be done about ageing, but it is possible to control the other risk factors associated with having a stroke.

Atherosclerosis

Atherosclerosis is the name given to the common problem of the hardening and furring up of the arteries. It can start at quite a young age when fatty streaks (atheroma) appear in the blood vessel wall. As people get older, these fatty streaks can cause sufficient damage to trigger the formation of a blood clot (thrombus) within the artery, leading to narrowing and a reduced blood flow. These blood clots can eventually block the blood vessel and cause a stroke if the artery leads to the brain. Most ischaemic strokes and TIAs are caused by these types of problems.

You can reduce your risk of atherosclerosis by altering your lifestyle. Eating a low-fat diet, with five portions of fresh fruit and vegetables daily, and taking regular exercise, will not only decrease the risk of atherosclerosis and help to reduce the risk of having a stroke, but will also protect against other circulatory problems, such as coronary heart disease and high blood pressure. It is particularly important to cut down on saturated fat, especially *trans*-fats, found in red meat and dairy products, because this type of fat increases the levels of blood cholesterol, a fatty substance that encourages blood clots to form.

Atherosclerosis

A coronary thrombosis occurs when a clot forms in the coronary arteries that supply blood to the heart muscle. In a heart attack a clot typically forms on a break in the fibrous plaque in a diseased vessel.

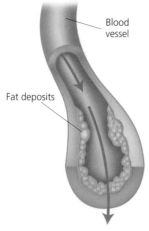

Blood vessel

Fat deposits

Fat deposits form on the walls of the artery

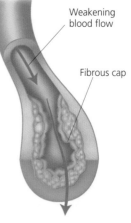

Weakening blood flow

Fibrous cap

Scar tissue forms a fibrous cap over the fat deposits

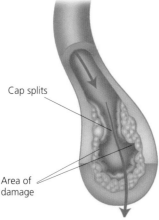

Cap splits

Area of damage

The cap is rigid and splits, creating a wider area of damage

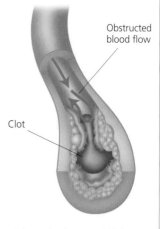

Obstructed blood flow

Clot

A large clot forms to seal the damaged area; this blocks the artery

High blood pressure

The medical term for high blood pressure is 'hypertension'. Most people know that hypertension is bad for you, but far fewer people realise that this is because the higher your blood pressure, the higher your risk of a stroke. When blood is forced through your circulatory system at high pressure, your artery walls receive a pounding. This damages the artery walls so that atherosclerosis and blood clots are more likely to occur.

Blood pressure is measured at two points in the heartbeat cycle. The highest pressure in the circulation occurs when the heart is contracting (the systolic pressure) and the lowest when the heart is at rest between beats (the diastolic pressure). This gives a

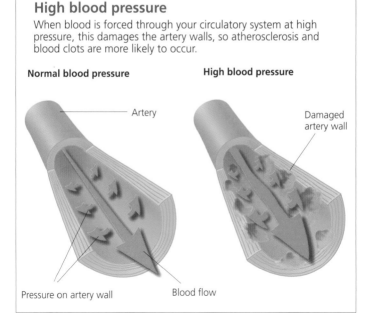

High blood pressure

When blood is forced through your circulatory system at high pressure, this damages the artery walls, so atherosclerosis and blood clots are more likely to occur.

Normal blood pressure   **High blood pressure**

Artery

Damaged artery wall

Pressure on artery wall   Blood flow

blood pressure measurement of two figures (systolic/diastolic), for example, 120/80. Researchers now know that, when your blood pressure rises and remains at a certain level, lowering your blood pressure will reduce your risk of a stroke. This is a rapidly changing subject at the moment, but most blood pressure experts would certainly want your blood pressure to be lower than 150/90.

Recent studies have indicated that it is variations in people's blood pressure rather than the average level that predicts stroke most powerfully and that occasional high values, and what might be called episodic hypertension, carry a high risk of stroke.

The latest recommendations consider a blood pressure below 140/85 to be ideal. For patients with diabetes or kidney impairment, or who already have cardiovascular disease, a target of below 130/80 is recommended. Some experts predicted that, if the average blood pressure could be lowered in the UK, there would be a dramatic reduction in the number of people who have strokes. Recent research from England and the USA suggests that this has indeed occurred, and as a result we are seeing a reduction in the expected numbers of strokes which, together with the ageing population, is keeping the total number of strokes seen about the same each year. This implies that stroke will be increasingly seen in frail elderly people, and become rarer in middle age.

Reducing your blood pressure

A high salt intake has been linked to high blood pressure. Salt increases blood pressure because it attracts fluid into the circulation, increasing the volume of blood, and reduces the amount of fluid lost through the kidneys. Some experts have suggested that some simple measures could dramatically reduce the stroke rate in the whole population. These measures include limiting the amount of salt in processed foods (for example, tinned soup) or labelling the salt content of all foods to allow consumers the chance to avoid salty foods.

Other methods of lowering blood pressure include stopping smoking, cutting down on alcohol and taking regular exercise. If all these methods fail, doctors can prescribe safe and effective blood pressure-lowering pills.

Unfortunately, high blood pressure often causes no symptoms and, even if your blood pressure is dangerously high, you may feel relatively well. It is therefore important to have your blood pressure checked regularly every year or so by your doctor or practice nurse as a routine part of health screening.

Smoking

Most people know that smoking is bad for their health, but many do not realise just how bad. Recent research has demonstrated that about half of all smokers will die prematurely from a smoking-related disease (for example, a heart attack, chronic bronchitis, a stroke, lung cancer). These odds of a premature death are considerably more than those for winning the national lottery. The good news is that stopping smoking improves your health almost immediately. You can probably halve your future risk of a stroke or a heart attack if you give up smoking. This is far better than any pill that your doctor could prescribe.

If you give up smoking, you will have much better health and also save money. Nicotine replacement therapy, such as patches or gum, can help you give up

Smoking

Smoking makes blood platelets 'stickier', so increasing the likelihood of blood clots forming in the circulation.

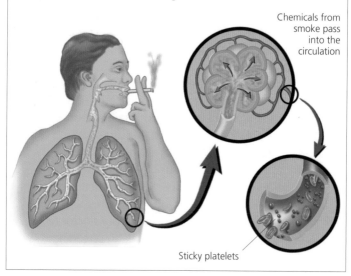

Chemicals from smoke pass into the circulation

Sticky platelets

smoking and are available without a prescription from pharmacies. Some people find that other methods such as hypnosis are also helpful.

Heart conditions

Atrial fibrillation is the most common heart problem known to increase the chances of having a stroke. It becomes more common as people get older and affects about 1 in 20 people aged over 65 years. It occurs when the heart beats irregularly, and increases the chance of blood clots forming in the heart. The blood clots can cause a stroke if they are carried by the circulation from the heart to the brain.

Treatment with the blood-thinning medication warfarin, or one of the newer anticoagulants, is the best

Common risk factors (causes) of a stroke

- Getting older
- High blood pressure
- Smoking
- Diabetes
- Heart trouble (for example, atrial fibrillation)
- Lack of exercise
- Blood disorders (for example, sickle cell disease)
- Excessive alcohol (for example, alcoholic binge drinking)

treatment for this problem because it will dramatically reduce the risk of a stroke. Aspirin is a simpler alternative to warfarin, but is not nearly as effective. If you notice that your heart rhythm has become irregular (for example, you experience palpitations), you should go to your doctor for a check-up.

Stroke in younger people

Although stroke is mainly a disease of elderly people, it can strike at any age, and is a particular tragedy for people under the age of 55 years. The diagnosis is often difficult because stroke is uncommon in this younger age group. The cause may be unusual and may mimic other complicated medical conditions. For this reason, an opinion from a neurologist (a specialist of diseases affecting the brain and nerves) is often very useful.

Causes of stroke in young people
Brain haemorrhages
A brain haemorrhage can occur at any age and can be responsible for the rare strokes that affect younger

people. Some haemorrhages – from, for example, a dilated weakening of an artery (aneurysm) that may have been present from birth – are so severe that they cause death in minutes or hours.

This sort of stroke is one of the causes of an unexpected death in a previously fit and healthy person. It often results in a sudden severe headache and collapse, leading to immediate coma. A CT (computed tomography) scan can confirm the diagnosis and patients will need specialised care in hospital. Surgery can be life saving for some patients, especially those with a bleed resulting from a cerebral aneurysm.

Heart problems

Some rare problems affecting the heart can cause stroke in younger people. These are generally conditions that cause blood clots to form in the heart, such as a congenital abnormality present from birth. Blood clots can cause strokes if they leave the heart and block an important blood vessel in the brain. If a young person has this type of stroke, he or she often needs to be assessed by a team of doctors, including a heart specialist.

Heart ultrasound scans (echocardiograms) involve placing a probe on the chest and may show a hole in the heart or another problem causing abnormal blood clots. Even better pictures can be obtained by placing the probe in the gullet (oesophagus). These scans are called TOEs, short for transoesophageal echocardiograms.

Damage to a blood vessel

Blood vessels in the neck can sometimes tear and split. This can cause a stroke if the vessels become blocked or abnormal blood clots are formed. The medical term for this problem is called a 'dissection'. The carotid artery

Echocardiography

An instrument called a transducer, which produces a beam of sound, is held against the chest. A picture of the heart is created by the reflected sound beams.

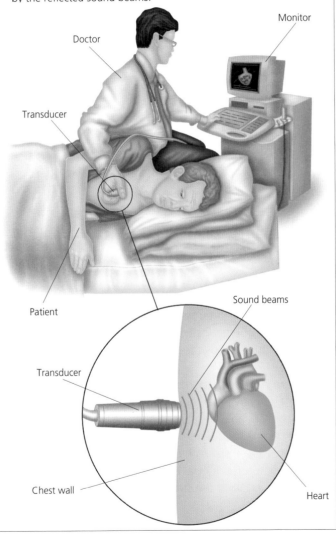

Monitor

Doctor

Transducer

Patient

Sound beams

Transducer

Chest wall

Heart

Risk factors for a stroke in people under 55

- Premature atherosclerosis
- Trauma
- Migraine
- Inflammatory conditions (for example, vasculitis)
- Systemic lupus erythematosus (SLE)
- Severe anaemia
- Alcoholic binge drinking
- Oral contraceptive pill
- Pregnancy
- Blood disorders
- Sickle cell anaemia*
- Protein C deficiency*
- Factor V Leiden disease (an inherited tendency to form blood clots)*
- Protein S deficiency*
- Platelet disorders
- Illegal recreational drugs (for example, cocaine)

*These conditions are all inherited disorders of blood clotting.

carries the main blood supply to the brain in the front of the neck. This artery can be damaged by trauma to the front of the neck such as attempted strangulation, sports injuries (rugby tackles) and car accidents.

Abnormal blood clotting
There are many inherited problems affecting blood clotting (see table above) but most of these are rare. Some people have a history of a number of medical problems as a result of blood clots (for example, deep vein thrombosis). Special blood tests are therefore useful, especially if the stroke has occurred before 35 years of age.

The pill

The oral contraceptive pill can cause a stroke in women, but the risk is very small. If 10,000 women take the pill for one year, on average one of these women will have a stroke as a result. These figures are based on the use of the combined pill, which includes an oestrogen and a progestogen. The risk is about three times that of a similar aged woman not on the pill. The risk appears to be higher if you smoke cigarettes.

Despite this threefold risk, the chance of a stroke is still tiny, because strokes are so rare during the child-bearing years. This risk is also small when compared with the usual risks of pregnancy. Overall, the benefits of the pill usually overwhelm the small increased risk of a stroke.

Hormone replacement therapy

Unfortunately, hormone replacement therapy (HRT) can cause similar problems to the contraceptive pill, with large clinical trials demonstrating the risks and benefits of treatment. The combined use of oestrogen and progesterone (for women with a uterus) and the use of oestrogen alone (for women who have had a hysterectomy) are both associated with a small increase in the risk of stroke.

HRT can carry additional risks (for example, pulmonary embolism) but also some benefits (for example, a reduction in bone fractures), so this subject is complicated and needs careful discussion with a doctor.

Illegal drugs

Recreational drugs, such as cocaine or ecstasy, or drugs used to enhance sports performance illegally can cause strokes in younger people. Unfortunately, an increasing number of drug-associated strokes are occurring and these are clearly avoidable disasters.

Migraine

Migraine is very common but still poorly understood. The symptoms of flashing lights and spreading abnormal sensations affecting the arms, face or legs are very common. Occasionally, these attacks can also be associated with temporary weakness. Very rarely, the migraine attack leaves a more permanent physical weakness called a migrainous stroke.

Rare inherited forms of strokes

Sometimes, a stroke in young adulthood may be caused by genetic problems, and one syndrome has recently been shown to run in families. It is very rare and causes multiple strokes. The syndrome has the name cerebral autosomal dominant arteriopathy with subcortical infarcts and leukoencephalopathy or CADASIL for short.

KEY POINTS

- Strokes become more common as people get older

- The major risk factors for stroke are high blood pressure, smoking and heart disease

- Dietary changes, such as cutting back on your salt intake and following a low-fat diet, may help to reduce your risk of a stroke

- In those aged under 55, stroke may be the result of unusual causes, such as a brain haemorrhage or recreational drugs

The stroke: what should you do?

You are having lunch with your grandmother when she suddenly slumps to one side. She is still conscious but doesn't seem to be able to talk, despite appearing to want to say something. The suddenness of the problem is characteristic of a stroke. What should you do?

Recognise the symptoms

You should know the signs of a stroke, as early diagnosis and treatment are vital in most cases. If the blood supply to part of the brain stops as a result of a stroke, the symptoms appear almost immediately and this gives the first major clue to the diagnosis.

The symptoms of a stroke may include: a sudden weakness or numbness of the face, arm or leg on one side of the body; sudden difficulty in speaking or understanding speech; and sudden blurring or a loss of vision (particularly in one eye).

The symptoms usually come on abruptly – within seconds for many people – and this is so unexpected that people can usually remember exactly what they were doing when the stroke came on. A stroke can also occur during sleep, and many people discover the stroke symptoms on waking up.

A useful reminder of the main symptoms of stroke as summarised in the FAST test:

F – Facial weakness: can the person smile? Has their mouth or eye drooped?
A – Arm weakness: can the person raise both arms?
S – Speech problems: can the person speak clearly and can they understand what they say?
T – Test all three symptoms, and if there any abnormalities dial 999 and ask for an emergency ambulance.

This test is increasingly used by paramedics in ambulance services to help get people with suspected stroke to hospital quicker because new stroke treatments have to be given very early after stroke onset to be beneficial.

Call for help
A stroke should be treated as a medical emergency and you should call for help immediately. Those involved in stroke medicine feel that speed is increasingly important in the assessment of a stroke. This is because some treatments offer the prospect of substantial benefit, but only if given very quickly.

Make sure that the person will not injure him- or herself (for example, by falling off a chair) and for most people calling an ambulance immediately on 999 is the best initial response. Although there may be some situations when hospital admission is inappropriate (for example, when a nursing home resident has an advanced care directive that specified comfort care in the event of a medical emergency) most people are best sent straight to hospital. When the ambulance arrives make sure that someone who witnessed the stroke travels with the patient, so that he or she can tell the hospital doctor on duty exactly what happened.

Going to hospital

Hospital care is needed for most patients with a stroke, and required urgently. On arrival at the hospital, the patient will be assessed in the accident and emergency department (or admission unit). A nurse will see the patient very soon after admission to note the severity of the problem and to alert the medical team. This nurse, called a triage nurse, makes sure that patients get the appropriate priority by assessing their health and determining how quickly they need to be treated. As some stroke treatments have to be given within minutes or a few hours of the stroke, people with stroke should be considered a high priority. In the past, patients with a stroke had not been considered a medical priority, but this is now changing with the implementation of stroke treatments such as thrombolysis (see page 46).

Patients who have had a suspected stroke will not normally be allowed to eat or drink until it has been confirmed that they have a safe swallow mechanism. Many patients with a stroke can choke if they are fed with fluids and food in the early stages. This swallowing difficulty usually recovers quickly.

Hospital diagnosis

When the hospital doctor assesses the patient, it is important to get a witnessed account (if available) from

Blood test

After a stroke, a blood test may be taken to help ascertain what caused it.

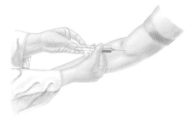

people who saw what happened. The doctor will ask several questions and then perform a full examination. Blood tests are taken to find out what caused the stroke and to look for abnormalities, such as too much sugar in the blood, which indicates diabetes. Diabetes is associated with abnormally high levels of glucose in the bloodstream, which hastens the onset of hardening and furring up of the arteries (atherosclerosis) and increases the risk of a stroke. If there is time to offer emergency treatment, the initial assessment will have to be quick, with a fast track to the stroke team and scanner.

The doctors need to assess which type of stroke has occurred: either a blood vessel has become blocked (an ischaemic stroke) or a blood vessel has burst (an intracerebral haemorrhage). To determine this, a brain scan has to be performed. The most widely used type of scan is the CT (computed tomography) scan, but a different technique, called magnetic resonance imaging (MRI), is an alternative. MRI gives a better cross-sectional image of soft tissues and does not use X-rays, so the patient is not exposed to radiation. These brain scans can show whether or not the stroke was caused by a bleed. If no blood is seen, doctors can be quite confident that the stroke has been caused by a blockage in the blood supply to the brain.

This information is very useful because future medical care depends on the stroke type. For example, blood-thinning treatment is not suitable for people whose stroke was caused by a bleed because this would make the bleeding worse. Newer MR scans can provide additional information to CT scanning, and are particularly useful in providing definite confirmation of a new stroke, especially if the CT scan appears normal.

Most patients will also have an electrocardiogram (ECG), which is a method of recording the electrical

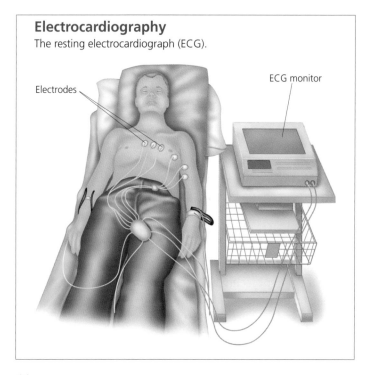

Electrocardiography
The resting electrocardiograph (ECG).

ECG monitor

Electrodes

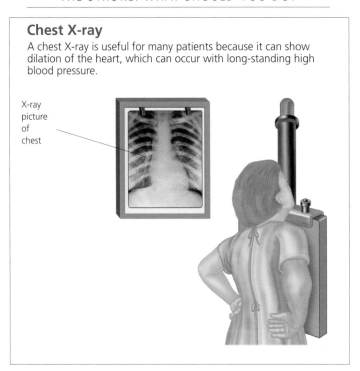

Chest X-ray

A chest X-ray is useful for many patients because it can show dilation of the heart, which can occur with long-standing high blood pressure.

X-ray picture of chest

activity of the heart by attaching wires to the chest, arms and legs. The ECG can show evidence of heart disease that may have caused the stroke. A chest X-ray may be useful later on but shouldn't delay early brain scanning. Chest X-rays can show dilation of the heart, which can occur with long-standing, untreated, high blood pressure, and may sometimes detect a dilated swelling (aneurysm) of the body's major artery, the aorta.

After the initial assessment and tests, the patient may have to be admitted to hospital. The main reasons for admission are to continue investigating the cause of the stroke, to give urgent treatment and to provide the

Magnetic resonance imaging (MRI)

Magnetic resonance imaging (MRI) uses powerful magnets to align the atoms in the part of the body being studied. Radiowave pulses break the alignment causing signals to be emitted from the atoms. These signals can be measured and a detailed image built up of the tissues and organs.

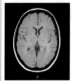

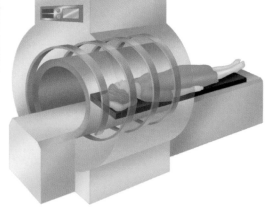

care needed if the stroke has caused some disability. One of the biggest revolutions in stroke medicine in the last 10 years has been research showing that organised stroke care (for example, stroke teams or units) can save lives and get more people back to their own home. As a result of this information, many health authorities are developing stroke units in major hospitals.

Immediate treatment

Exciting new treatments have been developed for acute stroke. Some treatments may now actually reverse the stroke, by dissolving the offending blood clot in the brain, leading to a complete recovery. Until recently, there was no effective pill or injection for a stroke, but

Computed tomography

Computed tomography (CT) fires X-rays through the brain at different angles. The X-rays are picked up by receivers and the information analysed by a computer to create a picture of the brain.

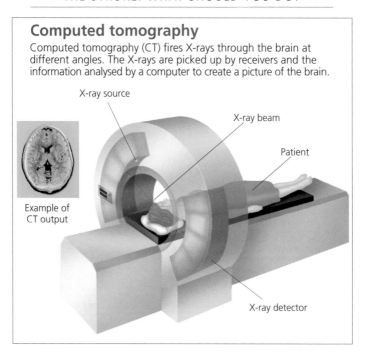

X-ray source

X-ray beam

Patient

Example of
CT output

X-ray detector

the last 20 years has seen a huge increase in stroke research. As a result of major clinical trials, some medicines have been shown to be very effective.

Thrombolytics

Thrombolytic treatment (or 'clot-busting' treatment) has been intensively studied for the past 15 years. It has been standard treatment for blocked blood vessels in the heart (to treat a heart attack) for many years, and is now the standard treatment for a blocked blood vessel in the brain (an ischaemic stroke). Clot-buster drugs dissolve the stringy protein (fibrin) that binds a clot together so that it breaks up. The treatment is given directly into a vein and must be given as soon as

Thrombolytics or 'clot busters'

Thrombolytic treatments (clot busters) dissolve the stringy protein (fibrin) that binds a clot together, so that it breaks up.

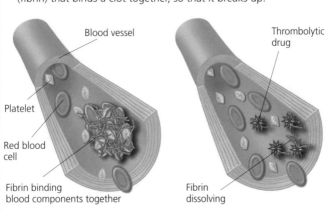

possible after the clot formed – and preferably within four to five hours.

Alteplase is the standard thrombolytic treatment in Europe and the good news is that hospitals in the United Kingdom are improving their ability to deliver this rather complicated treatment. Hospitals must have a stroke unit with a consultant stroke expert available and have access to brain scanning on a 24-hour basis. Stroke service provision is rapidly improving and in some areas, for example London, reorganisation of stroke services has been made to improve stroke thrombolysis delivery, with impressive increases in treatment rates. Treatment with alteplase is a powerful medical treatment and for every 100 people treated there will be about 10 to 15 more independent survivors.

Aspirin

Two large clinical trials have demonstrated that aspirin, in a dose of about 160 to 300 milligrams (mg) a day, is helpful for most people with a stroke. Before treatment, it is important for doctors to check that the stroke has not been caused by a bleed (as aspirin could make this worse) by performing an early brain scan. Aspirin works by reducing the stickiness of the blood cell fragments (platelets) that clump together to form a clot. It therefore reduces both the risk of a new clot forming and the chance of an early second stroke. It may even help stop the initial stroke getting worse.

Aspirin treatment is not very powerful. About 100 people need to be started on aspirin to prevent one death (or one person becoming disabled) in the first few weeks after the stroke. However, this very modest treatment benefit is worthwhile because aspirin is simple to take, has few side effects and is very cheap.

Aspirin

Aspirin works by reducing the stickiness of the small blood cells (platelets), which can clump together to form a clot.

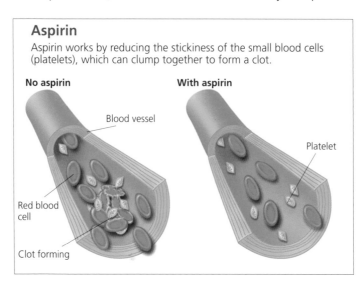

No aspirin

Blood vessel

Red blood cell

Clot forming

With aspirin

Platelet

Immediate aspirin treatment started in the early phase of stroke could save an estimated four lives a year in a single hospital alone (see 'Life after a stroke,' page 80). Put another way, the value of aspirin in the first two weeks after a stroke or TIA equals the benefit when taken for the next twelve months as secondary prevention.

Heparin and warfarin

These are both anticoagulant drugs. Anticoagulant drugs act by preventing the formation of the protein-based clotting factors that are essential for normal blood clotting. Warfarin has no immediate effect on existing blood clots because it takes two to three days to work. However, it can be used to prevent further blood clots in cerebral thrombosis and, therefore, to

---

Warfarin

Anticoagulant drugs (heparin and warfarin) act by preventing the formation of the protein-based clotting factors, which are essential for normal blood clotting.

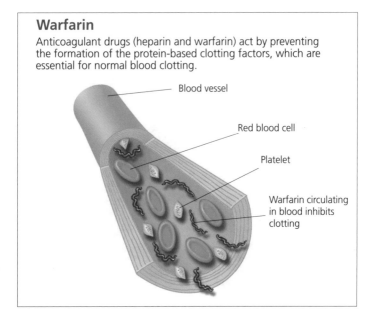

Blood vessel

Red blood cell

Platelet

Warfarin circulating in blood inhibits clotting

---

reduce the risk of a second stroke or TIA (see 'Life after a stroke', page 80). Heparin is now rarely used in stroke management or treatment because it has been shown to cause bleeding in the brain, triggering another stroke or haemorrhage.

Primary intracerebral haemorrhage

There are now promising new treatments emerging for stroke resulting from a brain haemorrhage. The blood-clotting agent (recombinant activated factor VII) has been tested in two major clinical trials with somewhat contradictory results so a larger confirmatory study will be required to establish the place of this treatment. Intensive blood pressure lowering is now also being tested with results expected in 2014.

Unfortunately, a trial of routine surgery to remove the brain haemorrhage was disappointing and neurosurgery is still applicable for only a small number of patients. A further trial investigating the role of more specialised neurosurgery is currently taking place. These new developments certainly help demolish the previous nihilistic approach to the treatment of stroke that was very prevalent a decade ago.

Randomised controlled trials

The above section has demonstrated the power of clinical trials in finding out new treatments for a previously untreatable condition. Further studies will be needed to improve stroke management. Therefore it is likely, and important, that many people with a stroke will, in the next few years, be asked to join a clinical trial.

People differ so much from each other, in so many ways, that doctors find it very difficult to predict who is going to do well (or badly) with a particular treatment. If the treatment is very new, enthusiastic doctors and their patients may think that the treatment is working, when in fact it is causing harm.

Over the last 50 years, scientists have developed a method of testing new medical treatments (or management strategies) called the randomised controlled trial. The idea behind this design is really quite straightforward. If the new treatment works, groups of people given the new treatment will do better than a similar group of people given the standard treatment.

As doctors are not very good at predicting who will do well and who will do badly, the two groups of patients are not chosen by the doctor but by a mathematical method called random allocation. Random allocation provides the best chance of creating two very similar groups of people. If all the people in one of these groups are then allocated the new treatment and these people, on average, do better than the group allocated the standard treatment, the difference is likely to be the result of the new treatment. Unfortunately, the randomised controlled trial is not foolproof because small trials can sometimes produce misleading results by the play of chance. It is a sobering thought that over 40,000 people with stroke had to be studied to identify the small benefit of aspirin for the acute stroke attack.

Consent and clinical trials

Doctors have to follow strict rules laid down by their local ethics committees when involving people in clinical trials. This protects the patient from unethical doctors. The most important part of the ethics of clinical trials is that patients understand that they are in a research trial and also the pros and cons of the different treatments under study. Not all good ideas work, but the design of clinical trials helps to reduce any unexpected hazard to a minimum.

To provide evidence that the researchers have explained the trial properly, patients usually sign a consent form. This can be difficult if the patient has just had a stroke because their thinking may not be clear or they may be unable to write or understand speech. Most ethics committees have agreed that a close relative (or perhaps even an independent person) can give permission if the patient is not in a position to do so. Some people have great concerns about this. However, a treatment for some types of strokes would never be found if a signed consent form was compulsory from everyone.

Most groups of experts and laypeople on ethics committees have therefore agreed that, under very strict conditions, some people with a stroke can be included in clinical trials, even if they are unable to give consent, provided that their family (or an independent expert) are happy with the project.

KEY POINTS

■ People should get urgent medical attention if they suddenly develop the symptoms of a stroke, even if the symptoms completely disappear

■ An early brain scan can help the doctors identify strokes caused by a brain haemorrhage

■ Clot-busting drugs, called thrombolytic therapy, are effective but only if given within a few hours from stroke onset. Specialised units are required to ensure that this complicated treatment is given to the correct people

■ Aspirin has a small but definite benefit for most people with a stroke, provided that the stroke is not caused by a bleed

■ More clinical trials will be needed to find the best treatment for a stroke

Stroke care

Hospital care

Most people having a stroke in the UK are admitted to hospital, and the first few days after admission are very busy. The patient is assigned a stroke team, a group of people who work together to ensure that the patient receives the relevant treatment and care. The doctors assess the severity of the stroke and organise tests.

One-stop clinics are currently being developed where all the tests, including a brain scan, are done on the same visit. The hospital doctor can then write a report to the GP, providing advice on how to manage the stroke once the patient has been discharged home. In many parts of the country, specialists for elderly people are able to visit elderly frail patients at home and advise on stroke management.

The nursing team make sure that the patient is comfortable and help with activities that are suddenly difficult. Physiotherapists, speech and language therapists, and occupational therapists also start their assessments to see what help each patient needs.

The stroke team
The doctors

Stroke medicine is a fairly new hospital specialty. The stroke specialist may be a geriatrician (a consultant for elderly people), a general physician or a neurologist (a consultant specialising in problems affecting the brain and nervous system). The hospital consultant usually works in a team with other consultants and junior doctors.

The doctor in charge will be the consultant. The doctor's role is to diagnose the stroke, organise the necessary tests and deal with medical complications. The doctor is also usually the team leader.

The nurses

The nursing staff provide the 24-hour care needed during the hospital stay. Nurses work in teams of fully qualified nurses (staff nurses), student nurses and care assistants (people who assist with patient care under the supervision of the staff nurses). The nurse in charge is now usually referred to as the charge nurse. In hospitals, there will always be nurses on the ward to help.

The nursing staff not only help with everyday activities such as washing, dressing and eating, but are also a source of information, advice and support. In many stroke units, they continue the work of the therapists on the ward.

The physiotherapist

The physiotherapy team concentrates on movement, posture and protection of vulnerable limbs, starting with basic abilities. Can the patient sit without support? If not, the therapist will advise the stroke team on the best positioning of the paralysed arms and legs, to avoid injuries and shoulder problems. As the person recovers, and gets stronger with therapy, the physiotherapist will concentrate on more complicated movements.

The work of physiotherapists is unique to every patient and is based on a thorough assessment and an individualised treatment regimen to restore normal movements. Great skill is needed to move people after a stroke and the physiotherapist works closely with the nursing staff to advise on the best method of moving people from beds to chairs and other 'transfers'. Some simple pieces of equipment such as a plinth, parallel rails and walking aids are needed and many therapists work in a gym as well as on the ward. There is a large amount of research evidence to demonstrate that physiotherapy can achieve a great deal, especially when specific tasks or activities are practised with a lot of repetition. There are concerns among many therapists

Physiotherapy

Even simple activities can be difficult after a stroke. In stroke units, physiotherapists concentrate on the following abilities (in order of difficulty):

- Sitting without help or support
- Standing for ten seconds
- Walking a few steps
- Walking ten metres
- Timed 10-metre walk (to improve speed and quality of walking)
- Climbing stairs

(Reproduced with permission from Mark Smith.)

that stroke patients do not get enough practice, even in stroke units. There are currently clinical trials taking place to establish exactly how intense or frequent activities should be.

The occupational therapist

The word 'occupation' refers to the 'skill of doing' many day-to-day tasks and activities that everyone takes for granted. These are often affected by a stroke and include managing to use the toilet, washing (and shaving), dressing, grooming (for example, combing hair), and making meals and drinks. These activities of daily living allow independence but perhaps not much quality of life. The extended activities of daily living allow a greater range of skills, and include using the telephone, shopping, leisure and hobbies, and using public transport and driving. Unfortunately, there is often little opportunity to work on these extended activities in the hospital system. In some areas, outpatient or domiciliary therapy can help people perform these more complicated tasks.

The speech and language therapist

The speech and language therapist will assess communication and swallowing problems. On admission, people with an acute stroke should have their swallowing assessed before being given any oral food, fluids or medication. This assessment can be very useful in adding to the neurological assessment of the stroke. Speech therapists have expanded their role in stroke care by becoming experts in the assessment of the swallowing mechanism. If swallowing is abnormal, they can try different types of foods to check the safest type of food for the patient. It is useful for them to continue to assess patients after a stroke, so that their diet can be modified as the stroke improves.

The more traditional role of the speech and language therapist is helping people to communicate if their speech and language have been affected by medical problems. People can be taught to say words more carefully so that they can be understood. This is often useful if the speech is very slurred (a problem called dysarthria). If the speech is very muddled after a stroke, this may mean that the person has lost the meaning of words or phrases, or cannot understand them. This is called dysphasia. An example of dysphasic speech is 'My sleg is very thratchy'; some words are correct but are not the right ones, other words appear to be nonsense. In this example, the person was trying to tell a doctor about his uncomfortable compression stockings. Speech and language therapists can help patients to cope with these problems. Various charts and pictures can help with everyday communication with nursing staff and carers.

Social worker

A stroke can affect all aspects of life, and there are many services and financial resources available. The social worker is the expert in the resources available locally and the types of financial benefits that you might be able to claim. He or she is therefore a vital part of the stroke team when the time is right to plan a discharge back home, or when alternatives have to be considered. Some people may manage with a home help twice a week, whereas others may need a complex package of care, including community nurses, carers visiting four times a day and day care in stroke clubs.

Many services are now means tested (the cost depends on the patient's financial situation). If the patient has sufficient resources, he or she may need to contribute financially to the care; if not, the local council social services department will be responsible. This can be a very complicated area indeed, and the social worker's role is crucial in planning a successful discharge from the hospital.

Team work

Rehabilitation is focused on individual patients. The team will get to know an individual's needs, aspirations and family circumstances. It usually meets each week and every team member reports to the group. The team considers whether people are achieving their goals and the likely outcome is predicted. Most rehabilitation teams continue to work with patients until they are fit to return home.

Unfortunately, some people do not recover enough to get back home, even with maximum care in the community. When this looks likely, it is important for the hospital team to discuss this with the patient and their family (or main carers). Complicated or difficult situations sometimes need to be discussed at meetings attended by the patient, the family and the stroke team (these are sometimes called family conferences). The team can hear the detailed wishes of the family, and the family can be updated on any progress.

The first few days
Getting comfortable and protecting your body

It is very easy for patients to hurt themselves shortly after a stroke. Their muscles are often weak and their muscles and tendons are easily damaged through lying awkwardly, trying to move about or accidents such as a fall. Shoulder problems cause the greatest trouble. The stroke team will teach the patient the best way to sit in a chair and lie in bed. Correct positioning will also protect the arms, shoulders and legs of someone with a recent stroke from pressure that may lead to a strain or bed sores.

Walking

If the patient cannot walk after a stroke, he or she will be confined to a bed or chair while the physiotherapists advise on the best way to manage movement. During the early stages of a stroke, many patients are allowed to walk only if they are supervised by the physiotherapist. This is to avoid practising walking methods that may be bad for some patients. For some, it can be better to delay walking until they are strong enough to walk with a normal pattern of movement.

The increased spasticity of the stroke-affected limbs needs to be controlled, and this is often the main focus of early rehabilitation (see 'Types of strokes', page 14). Physiotherapists may spend a great deal of time getting the patient to relax and to reduce the disabling stiffness of the affected limbs. Some patients try to walk at too early a stage in their rehabilitation. It is important to realise that practising 'undesirable' movements may delay or complicate the best recovery after a stroke. Great patience is needed by everyone at this stage.

Eating

Swallowing problems are very common after a stroke. The basic problem is that both food and air have to use the mouth. Normally, the body makes sure that the air goes to the lungs and the food goes down to the

Swallowing problems

Swallowing problems are very common after a stroke. The basic problem is that both air and food have to pass through the mouth to reach the lungs and stomach.

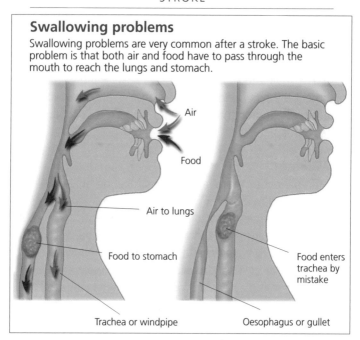

Air

Food

Air to lungs

Food to stomach

Food enters trachea by mistake

Trachea or windpipe

Oesophagus or gullet

stomach. This complex process is often disturbed in the early stages of a stroke, and can lead to problems if food goes down the wrong tube and damages the lungs or causes a chest infection. To help prevent early chest infections, the stroke team will usually test the ability of the patient to swallow a test drink of water. If there is doubt about the safety of the swallow mechanism, patients will be given no food or drink (called 'nil by mouth') and a further, more detailed, assessment will be needed.

Speech and language therapists have taken a leading role in assessing whether people can swallow or not, although this may be done by other members of the stroke team. If people are unable to swallow food or water safely, there are various alternative methods of maintaining essential fluids and food. Simple fluids can be given into a vein or into the skin (intravenous or subcutaneous routes). Food and drink can be given by a tube placed into the stomach through the nose or directly into the stomach through the skin.

In the first week of stroke it is possible to feed people with a nasogastric tube and this treatment may prevent some patients from dying as a result of their stroke, but, unfortunately, this feeding method does not improve longer-term independent survival. In the first month after a stroke, if patients do not recover their swallowing ability, a nasogastric feeding tube is best, but for longer-term use (months or years) a tube placed straight into the stomach (called a PEG tube for short) is the most practical option. These feeding decisions can be very difficult for patients and their families to make and may require repeated discussion with the stroke team.

Urine and bowels

Many people with a stroke are unable to use the toilet independently and this causes understandable distress. Passing urine and opening the bowels are private activities, and it is a great shock to have to depend on others for the first time for many decades. Although many people with a stroke maintain full control, others become incontinent for a while.

The occasional accident is sometimes unavoidable because people may get too little warning to ask for help in time. Fortunately, the stroke team are aware of these problems, and most people can be helped back to full independence. In the initial stages, patients may have to ask for help each time that they need to use the toilet. Bottles and commodes at the bedside may be required for some people. To cope with the immediate problem, some people need a urinary catheter, which is a tube placed into the bladder to drain the urine.

Stroke rehabilitation units

Just under half of all strokes are mild and patients have little or minimal disability, little or no difficulty with speech or swallowing, and no loss of consciousness. There is then no need to keep people in hospital unless further investigations are needed. Many people with mild strokes can therefore be managed at home, or can be discharged from the hospital within a week or so.

Unfortunately, about a third of people with a stroke have significant problems with everyday activities and need a great deal of help. Such strokes are thus called moderate or severe strokes. Although rehabilitation at home is possible, it can be very expensive and difficult to coordinate and most people disabled after a stroke will be admitted to hospital.

The stroke team will usually be able to predict who is going to need continued rehabilitation during the first week or two of hospital care. Stroke rehabilitation facilities vary widely. In some hospitals, people with a stroke are transferred to a stroke rehabilitation unit, which may or may not be on the same site. In other hospitals, people are cared for on 'general medical' or 'care of elderly people' wards. Despite these different types of wards, the rehabilitation process is similar. The aim of stroke rehabilitation is to get patients back to normal life as soon as possible, with the minimum disruption to them and their family.

Rehabilitation depends on good team work. With so many health workers involved, it is immediately obvious that good communication is important. Every stroke is different and every rehabilitation programme needs to be designed to suit the individual. A key part of rehabilitation is good initial assessment of the problems by each member of the team and a plan of how to overcome each problem.

The good news about strokes is that most people improve over time as the swelling resolves and different parts of the brain learn to take over some of the functions carried out by brain cells that have been damaged or destroyed. The natural recovery can be quite dramatic for some. Most of the improvement occurs in the first three months, but further recovery can occur even later. A common phrase used is: 'a stroke comes on quickly, most people improve, but improvement can be slow.' During this period of natural recovery, stroke rehabilitation has been shown to be very effective.

Returning home

It is quite common for patients to need several months of rehabilitation in hospital, especially when the stroke has caused more severe disability. The thought of getting home can therefore be a major source of worry to both the patient and his or her family. Will they cope? Will there be problems? Stroke teams help solve these worries by a variety of different approaches.

Home visit assessment

The home visit assessment is very useful for people recovering from a stroke. Before a planned discharge from hospital, the therapists (usually the occupational therapist and physiotherapist) take the patient home for the day, together with the key family members, and check that they are going to manage. Very simple problems may be found. For example, the steps into the house may need to be altered. Rails at doorways and in halls may be useful. Bathroom equipment is often required, for example, a raised toilet seat or a shower chair.

The therapists ask patients to do everyday tasks, such as get out of bed, go to the toilet or make a meal in their own kitchen. They can then report back to the stroke team with their recommendations. Things may have gone so well that an immediate discharge can be planned. At other times, more time may be needed to allow further preparation.

Occasionally, the home visit assessment confirms major problems that are not so easily overcome. In this situation, alternatives to going home will need to be explored.

When a return home is not possible

In many areas, particularly the more urban areas of the UK, it is possible to get back home even if the stroke has left moderate-to-severe disabilities (for example, unable to walk). This is made possible by regular carers who come into the home and help. The stroke team may plan quite complicated packages of care for some patients. These community care packages can help avoid nursing home care but are dependent on local facilities and funding. Not all areas can provide such comprehensive care, especially for more rural parts.

For some patients it is simply not possible to look after them in their own home and alternatives have to be considered. Residential and nursing homes are particularly useful for people who have become confused or require 24-hour care.

Residential homes

These homes are staffed 24 hours a day by care assistants. Each resident has his or her own room (or shared room). All the meals are provided, together with a laundry service and room cleaning, and staff are available to guide residents. Residents must be mobile and continent (or able to manage their own catheters or pads). This type of home is useful for very frail people and those who may have some degree of dementia and therefore need guidance and prompting. Although some of these homes are council run, many have been privatised. In the UK, the fees for these homes will depend on where you live (the rules in Scotland are slightly different to those in the rest of the UK) and your personal circumstances.

Your social worker will advise you on these complex matters. You may have to contribute to the cost of your care. If you are funding the residential home yourself, the costs can be considerable and can vary depending on the facilities available. Generally, the patient's family would choose the residential home, with advice from the social worker. If the patient has no immediate family or friends available, the social worker can help the patient choose the best home. Visits to view such homes, before a definitive decision, can be very useful and many patients often meet old friends, especially if a local home is identified.

Nursing homes

Nursing homes differ from residential homes because they always have state-registered nurses on duty on a 24-hour basis. These homes are therefore useful if you need help with personal care (for example, going to the toilet, washing, dressing) or have more complicated nursing needs, such as tube feeding, regular turning in bed (to avoid pressure sores) or dressings to skin wounds. Some people are required to contribute to the nursing home fees. In general, these contributions are to cover the costs of providing the room, laundry, catering and cleaning, the so-called 'hotel' costs. These additional contributions are means tested, and will therefore depend on the financial assessments completed by your social worker. The nursing homes are usually chosen by the family. The social worker can provide a list of locally approved homes. These homes are more expensive than residential homes.

The social workers can provide extremely useful financial advice for patients who are moving into residential or nursing home care because most patients should receive extra government support even if they have money of their own (for example, attendance allowance).

NHS continuing care

There are still some NHS-run hospital nursing homes (long-term care) available in parts of the country. These units usually have a doctor visiting regularly and a consultant geriatrician visiting each week. These facilities are useful for people with very complicated nursing or medical needs. For example, if patients need intravenous fluids from time to time, or have other medical problems that require frequent attention. These units are currently considered as part of the NHS and are therefore free of charge.

KEY POINTS

■ All people with suspected stroke should, if possible, be admitted immediately to a specialised stroke unit

■ The first few days in hospital are very busy as each member of the medical team starts his or her assessments

■ The ability to swallow food and liquid can be disturbed after a stroke and this needs special attention

■ Stroke rehabilitation improves independence after a stroke and increases the number of people able to return home

■ Before being discharged from hospital, you may be taken for an assessment visit to check that you will manage

■ Unfortunately, some people are too disabled to manage at home and alternatives have to be considered

Complications after a stroke

Strokes affect many older people, and other common medical conditions, such as heart disease, diabetes or arthritis, are often associated with a stroke. In addition, there are a few conditions that complicate recovery after having a stroke. These are some of the more common problems encountered.

Depression

Depression is quite common after a stroke, and affects about a fifth of people in the recovery phase. A stroke is a shock to the system and many people suffer losses (for example, of mobility and independence) as a result. The person may need to be admitted to hospital, which can be upsetting, and many patients find that their whole life is totally transformed by the stroke event. Feelings of depression are a natural reaction to this, and sometimes the depression becomes severe enough to need treatment.

The symptoms of depression include low mood, crying, low self-esteem and feelings of hopelessness. Sometimes, depression can affect the appetite, and people simply cannot be bothered to prepare food or eat it. Many of these symptoms, when mild, are a normal part of life, but, when severe, they can cause misery and stop or slow recovery. There is no clear dividing line between low mood and depression, and the doctor will often judge when the symptoms will benefit from treatment with an antidepressant drug.

Many different types of antidepressants are available, but the treatment takes time to start working (perhaps two to three weeks) and needs to be continued for months (six months or more). Support from the stroke team is also important for people with depression.

Emotional changes

Many people experience a change in their emotions after a stroke, because the emotional centres of their brain may have been affected, or the changes that they have experienced may upset them. Some people find that they suddenly burst into tears for no apparent reason, and this type of reaction can continue for several weeks or months and occasionally longer. If this tearfulness is associated with depression, it should respond to antidepressants and, even in the absence of depression, this type of drug can help if the reaction causes distress.

Epilepsy

Epilepsy is an excessive electrical activity of brain cells that triggers a seizure. Seizures can vary from short lapses in consciousness to severe spasms of the whole body, and some people develop more than one type of fit. A stroke is the most common cause of epilepsy occurring for the first time in older people. It is thought to occur as a result of damage to electrical circuits in the brain or the formation of scar tissue. About five per cent (one in twenty) of patients will have an epileptic fit after a stroke. These fits may require treatment, especially if they recur.

Chest infections

Chest infections can occur after a stroke, especially if the swallow mechanism has been affected. This makes inhalation of food particles more likely, so that inflammation and infections occur. Symptoms include a cough, a high temperature and breathlessness. Most chest infections can be treated with a simple course of antibiotics. Chest physiotherapy and breathing exercises are also helpful.

Urinary tract infections

A stroke may affect the ability to pass urine, so that the bladder does not empty fully, making infections more common. Stinging or scalding on passing urine may occur, but often the infections go unnoticed by the patient. A short course of antibiotics can treat a urine infection, and nursing care together with good hygiene can reduce the chance of it recurring.

Painful shoulder

The shoulder joint is only as strong as its surrounding muscles. These muscles are often weak after a stroke, and the tendons and muscles are easily damaged. Pain may occur in the first few hours and days after a stroke through lying awkwardly, when trying to move about or through accidents such as a fall. Skilled handling by physiotherapists, occupational therapists and nursing staff can often prevent this distressing problem and, if it occurs, physical treatments (provided by physiotherapists) are often better than painkillers prescribed by doctors.

Dementia

Stroke disease is the second most common cause of dementia after Alzheimer's disease. This is particularly important if patients have had a number of strokes. Although problems with memory and the intellect after stroke have been recognised for many years, this area has been neglected by many doctors and researchers. Specialists for elderly people (geriatricians) and psychiatrists for elderly people (psychogeriatricians) may be able to provide advice on management and access to local services such as a day hospital or respite support. Occasionally, a stroke can cause very abnormal behaviour, which requires specialised psychiatric nursing and medical care, and medication to control difficult behaviour.

Pain

Sometimes the stroke affects the pain pathways in the brain, and pain becomes a problem. The pain is often described as being a 'deep' pain, a 'toothache-type pain' in the bones and muscles of the arm or leg. It tends to follow the same pattern as the weakness after stroke (see 'Types of strokes', page 14). This type of pain is often difficult to treat, but various painkillers are available to give some relief.

Case history

A 60-year-old man had a stroke causing a weakness down his left arm and left leg. As the weakness improved, he developed a deep pain in his arm and thigh. Simple painkillers didn't help and, after several weeks of discomfort, the doctors found a tablet that took the edge off the pain. This treatment was not a normal painkiller. It was a drug usually used for epilepsy that seems to dampen down the way that electrical pain messages are passed along nerves.

Thrombosis

Thrombosis is the name given to abnormal blood clots. After a stroke, people are at an increased risk of a blood clot lodging in their leg (deep vein thrombosis). Movement is important to keep the blood flowing through the leg muscles properly. After a stroke, immobility means that the blood flow through the legs is more sluggish than usual, so clots are more likely to form.

Less commonly, a blood clot can travel from where it formed in the deep veins to obstruct the blood flow in the lungs. This type of wandering blood clot is called an embolus, and a clot lodging in the lungs is known as a pulmonary embolism (pulmonary is the medical word relating to the lungs). A pulmonary embolism can be a serious complication and may be fatal, because it can prevent enough blood reaching the lungs to receive all the oxygen that the body needs. Fortunately, this is rare, and the rate of a fatal lung thrombosis is probably less than one in a 100 of those with disabling stroke. The symptoms of a pulmonary embolism include sudden breathlessness, palpitations, faintness and chest pain on breathing.

Pulmonary embolism

Thrombosis is the name given to abnormal blood clots. After a stroke people are at an increased risk of a blood clot lodging in their legs. A blood clot that moves in the body is called an embolus, and a clot that lodges in the blood vessels in the lungs is called a pulmonary embolism.

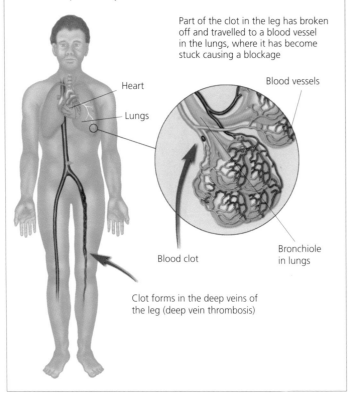

Part of the clot in the leg has broken off and travelled to a blood vessel in the lungs, where it has become stuck causing a blockage

Heart

Lungs

Blood vessels

Bronchiole in lungs

Blood clot

Clot forms in the deep veins of the leg (deep vein thrombosis)

Researchers suspect that deep vein thrombosis and embolism are becoming less common with the modern emphasis on early rehabilitation and early mobilisation after a stroke. Blood-thinning treatments, such as aspirin and heparin, can be life saving because they thin the blood and help to dissolve the clot.

Support stockings

Compression stockings squeeze the superficial veins in the leg, forcing blood to flow through the deep veins and preventing the pooling of blood associated with clot formation.

Without compression stockings

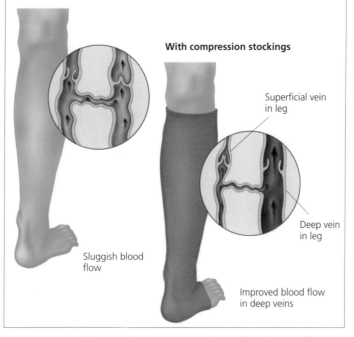

With compression stockings

Superficial vein in leg

Deep vein in leg

Sluggish blood flow

Improved blood flow in deep veins

However, although heparin can reduce the chance of developing a leg thrombosis, it can increase the chance of abnormal bleeding in the brain. Special elastic leg stockings (compression stockings) were commonly used to prevent deep vein thrombosis but a recent trial, the CLOTS study, demonstrated that they didn't significantly reduce thrombosis and were definitely causing skin side effects such as ulcers, so this method is going out of favour. Other physical methods are now being tested.

Dying after a stroke

A stroke is the third most common cause of death in the UK. This is mainly as a result of a stroke affecting older people, many of whom already have other serious medical problems. After a stroke, about 10 per cent of people (1 in 10) die within a week, 20 per cent within a month and 30 per cent within a year. About a fifth of people admitted to hospital will die as a direct result of their stroke.

Most people die very peacefully after a major stroke and are not in any pain or discomfort. Some strokes are so severe that they cause immediate coma. Death occurs when the brain is no longer able to keep the body breathing or the circulation flowing. This results from the effect of the stroke on a part of the brain called the brain stem, which means that the person drifts into a deeper and deeper coma and eventually dies.

Occasionally, people survive in a coma for a few weeks (or even longer), and this period can be very distressing for the family and stroke team. There is often the dilemma of what to do about feeding the patient. Some patients appear more comfortable without feeding tubes or intravenous or subcutaneous drips. But some families become very distressed at the thought of not feeding someone and, of course, this will always lead to death. If there is genuine uncertainty about the degree of recovery, it is often wiser to continue some fluid and nutritional support. There are no easy answers, and it is often best to discuss these issues with the stroke team.

If the stroke has caused so much brain damage that the patient has been in a coma for more than a few days, he or she may not recover and the treatment should aim to keep him or her comfortable. Good nursing care is required, ideally in a quiet, well-lit environment with privacy for the family. Sometimes, giving the patient fluid (via a drip) can appear to help, but on other occasions this treatment can cause swelling (oedema) of the legs and arms. The question of whether to give fluid will therefore depend on the state of the patient and avoiding fluids can actually be a positive decision. Despite good nursing care and nutritional support, most patients in a coma after a stroke die within days or weeks of their stroke.

Deaths after a stroke are often not the result of the direct effects of the stroke on the brain but of the complications of becoming disabled. These complications include chest or urinary infections and thrombosis affecting the lungs (pulmonary embolism).

'Do not resuscitate' orders

If someone is admitted to hospital after a stroke, there is usually a cardiac resuscitation team in the hospital to try to save lives in the event of a cardiac or respiratory arrest (when the heart or breathing stops). Unfortunately, the success rate is not good for many patients and prolonged resuscitation often causes brain damage. Doctors may decide that resuscitation is so unlikely to succeed that it is best avoided for some people. In this situation, they may recommend a 'Do not resuscitate' order. If the doctors feel that a patient may benefit from resuscitation, the patient may be asked for his or her views on this. Some people do not want resuscitation and have strongly held views on the matter. Do not be alarmed if this subject is mentioned during the hospital stay, because it is increasingly common to obtain the views of patients and relatives on these difficult ethical decisions.

KEY POINTS

■ A number of complications can occur after a stroke; many can be prevented by organised stroke care and most can be successfully treated

■ Strokes are the third most common cause of death in the UK

■ Most deaths are peaceful, with patients drifting into a coma in the final few hours or days

Life after a stroke

A stroke can have a dramatic effect on someone's life, but many people recover and return home. Sometimes, patients feel abandoned after being discharged from the stroke clinic or day hospital. Fortunately, there are excellent services provided by the voluntary and charity sectors. Many of these charities offer a range of leaflets, help and advice, and clubs and activity groups, as well as family support officers. Their contact details are listed in 'Useful addresses' (page 107).

Mood changes

Some families note a slight change in the person's personality or mood. This is not surprising because these parts of behaviour are controlled by the brain, which is affected by a stroke. A stroke can cause depression or anxiety, and anyone who has either of these should be encouraged to see his or her GP.

Sometimes after a stroke, people can experience mood swings and outbursts, such as crying for no apparent reason. They may also show their frustration at their slow rate of recovery. These changes may improve after a few months, but sometimes they can be permanent.

Hobbies and activities

For some people, it is impossible to return to their usual activities, because of problems that remain after the stroke. Others are nervous about returning to their usual activities and some are too frightened to restart hobbies or interests. People need to be reassured that their activities will not bring on another stroke, and it is important to increase activities, as recovery allows, to return to as normal a life as possible. There are no major rules to follow (apart from the driving laws) and barriers should not be placed in the way of someone trying to get back to normal.

Case history

A retired hospital consultant had a major stroke requiring six months' rehabilitation. He was eventually discharged to his upstairs flat. The provision of a chair lift allowed him to visit his garden and he continued to get great pleasure from supervising his wife at work!

Sexual intercourse

Resuming sexual activity following recovery from stroke is usually safe. However, if your stroke was caused by a bleed, you should consult your GP. Sexual sensations are often not affected by a stroke, but couples may need time to adapt to their new circumstances, especially if they have been left with disabilities. If problems occur, your family doctor can help to identify any obvious medical problem. The Stroke Association can also provide you with information and advice (see 'Useful addresses', page 117).

Case history

A 60-year-old woman was attending the day hospital because of problems with recurrent urinary incontinence. Despite a great deal of effort by the nurses and doctors, they were unable to improve the problem and a permanent urinary catheter was recommended. The patient was determined to avoid a catheter at all costs and, on further discussion, this was because she did not want 'a tube' to interfere with her sexual activity.

None of the day hospital staff had asked about sexual activity and had not realised that she enjoyed regular intercourse with her husband. It is easy for medical staff to assume incorrectly that sexual activity stops with increasing age (or after a stroke).

Driving after a stroke

In the UK, the responsibility for informing the Driver and Vehicle Licensing Agency (DVLA) rests with the patient and not the doctor. If a person has had a stroke or transient ischaemic attack (TIA), with symptoms lasting more than a month, he or she has a statutory requirement to write to the DVLA and let them know. The address is: Drivers Medical Unit, DVLA, Swansea SA99 1TU.

If there is any doubt about a person's fitness to drive, it is possible to undergo a special assessment by driving occupational therapists, who are able to check driving skills and write a report for the DVLA. If a person has an accident despite being told not to drive their car, their insurance will not be valid and they will not be insured.

Driving restrictions

The following section we believe to be correct at time of publication, but readers are advised to make their own enquiries to confirm that this is still the case, because the situation may have subsequently changed.

After a stroke or a single TIA, people must not drive for a month. At one month, it may be possible for the person to restart driving if they have made a good recovery from the stroke, that is, the stroke has not caused problems with muscle control, eyesight, coordination or *memory* or *understanding*. It is probably wise for people to get advice from their doctor about this. Any large problem in field of vision that remains after a stroke is a bar to driving. If people have frequent TIAs (for example, several attacks a week for a while), they must not drive for three months, and it is very important to get medical advice.

There are more restrictive rules for people who make their living by driving (for example, drivers of large goods vehicles or LGVs or passenger-carrying vehicles or PCVs). These rules are there to protect the public and the driver. For those with vocational driving licences who have a stroke, they may lose the vocational driving licence and, by implication, their job. Their doctors and employers will need to advise them on the rules for their particular circumstances.

Seizures after a stroke

If someone had a fit (also called a seizure) at the start of a stroke (within the first 24 hours), but no subsequent fits, he or she should not drive for one month (the same rules as for a stroke) and should inform the DVLA (see above). If he or she has a fit later on in the recovery period, the person should not drive for 12 months. It may be possible in the future to get a driving licence if the fits can be completely controlled, but specialist advice is recommended for this situation.

Case history

A 70-year-old man had problems with his memory and intellect (early dementia) after a stroke. He asked his hospital consultant for permission to return to driving. The consultant established that the patient had adequate vision and strength in his muscles, but was concerned about the mild dementia. The consultant advised that he should not drive. The patient was unhappy with that decision and a formal occupational therapy driving assessment was arranged. The driving test was a disaster, with the patient consistently driving into the kerb. The therapist confirmed that the patient should not drive; he accepted the decision and the DVLA revoked the driving licence.

Preventing a second stroke

It is generally true that the risk of a second stroke is much greater than for someone who has never had a stroke. This means that prevention becomes much more important. In the year after a first stroke, the risk of another stroke (if stroke preventive medications are not taken) is about ten per cent, or one in ten. This is about ten times the risk of a similar person who has never had a stroke. In the following years, the risk, without treatment, is lowered to about five per cent, or one in twenty. These estimates are true for most types of stroke. The good news is that lifestyle changes and medication can substantially lower these risks.

To prevent a second stroke, patients may need to modify their lifestyle. In some cases, they may also be prescribed drugs or require surgery. The best methods of preventing a further stroke depend on the type of stroke previously experienced. It is therefore important to know whether the stroke was caused by a bleed in the brain (a primary intracerebral haemorrhage) or a blockage in the blood supply (an ischaemic stroke or cerebral infarct).

Lifestyle changes

There is plenty that stroke patients can do themselves to prevent a second stroke or even prevent a first stroke. For details of how your lifestyle increases your risk of a stroke, see 'Why have you had a stroke?' (page 26). Self-help measures to reduce the risk of a stroke include:

- stopping smoking
- eating a healthy, low-fat, low-salt diet
- losing excess weight
- taking regular exercise (once given the medical go-ahead)
- good control of diabetes if present, with a healthy diet, medication if necessary and regular monitoring of blood glucose levels
- reducing alcohol intake to within safe limits
- stopping oral contraceptives in younger women
- regular blood pressure checks.

Blood-thinning treatments

In the case of an ischaemic stroke, the next step to consider is a blood-thinning treatment to prevent future blood clots. These treatments include antiplatelet drugs and anticoagulants. The most commonly used antiplatelet drug is aspirin. The most commonly used anticoagulant is warfarin, which is more potent than aspirin in thinning the blood. Heparin is not usually used, because it has been associated with bleeding in the brain early after stroke and has to be given by injection. There are many new anticoagulants that will probably replace warfarin over the next decade. After a stroke caused by a bleed (primary intracerebral haemorrhage), patients should avoid medicines that thin the blood.

Aspirin

Aspirin has been used as a medical treatment for decades. In addition to helping with rheumatic-type pain and headaches (in large doses), it has long been known to thin the blood by making part of the blood (the platelets) less sticky (in small doses). Overall, aspirin has been shown to reduce the chance of blood clots for many conditions, and is now the standard treatment for heart attacks and most types of stroke.

Aspirin has side effects, like all drugs, and these include indigestion, as a result of aspirin's effect on the stomach. This can sometimes cause bleeding in the gut, which can occasionally be serious. Aspirin must therefore be taken regularly only on the advice of a doctor. The side effects can be reduced by using a very low daily dose (only a tiny amount of aspirin seems to be required). A dose of as low as 30 milligrams (mg) a day may be effective, but doses of between 75 and 300 mg a day are equally effective and are the sorts of doses generally used in the UK. Recent evidence has suggested that aspirin may have additional benefits in reducing the risk of cancers, but this observation will need confirmation in further studies.

Other antiplatelet drugs

There are now other medicines available that can also make the blood less sticky through an antiplatelet effect. These treatments include dipyridamole, clopidogrel and ticlopidine. These newer treatments have been the subject of much research. Clopidogrel is a useful alternative to aspirin, if the patient is intolerant of aspirin.

Recent work has concentrated on studying combinations of antiplatelet drugs and the combination of aspirin and clopidogrel has been found to be beneficial if taken for a few months after a heart attack, but was not beneficial if taken after a stroke. In contrast, the combination of aspirin and dipyridamole has been found to be an effective combination for people who have a normal heart rhythm after an ischaemic stroke. The main drawback to this particular combination is that some people do not tolerate the dipyridamole because of headache or gastrointestinal symptoms. It has been found that, if people do get headaches when starting this new combination, a few doses of paracetamol usually help and the headaches resolve in a few days.

Anticoagulants

Warfarin is the most widely used anticoagulant, but this will change in the next few years as newer agents become more widely used. Warfarin is a naturally occurring compound that makes the blood less sticky. It stops the formation of blood clots. The main role of warfarin is to thin the blood in people with a medical condition that causes abnormal blood clots.

The most important heart condition associated with blood clots causing strokes is the condition called atrial fibrillation (AF). In this condition, part of the heart beats abnormally, giving rise to an irregular heart beat. The two atria beat irregularly, and often at a rate of 100 beats per minute or more. This causes the ventricles to beat at a similar (or lower) rate. Overall the heart pump is out of sync – the sequence of the beat is disturbed and the pulse feels erratic. This abnormality is associated with an increased risk of having a stroke because blood clots are more likely to form within the heart, from where they can travel up to the brain. If patients have this heart problem and have had a stroke caused by a blocked blood vessel, warfarin treatment is much better than aspirin, provided that patients can tolerate warfarin.

Unfortunately, the decision to use warfarin can be difficult. The effective dose varies from person to person and also from time to time. Frequent blood tests (called the INR or international normalised ratio) are needed when warfarin is first started and then regular blood tests (perhaps once a month) are needed while treatment is continued. Warfarin can cause abnormal bleeding and therefore people who have a bleeding problem (for example, regular nose bleeds or a previous major bleed in the brain or gut) should avoid warfarin.

Warfarin interacts with many other medicines and should not be taken with aspirin. It can even interact with paracetamol. If people have trouble reading medicine labels, fall a great deal or get confused, warfarin treatment can be quite risky. Despite these difficulties, tens of thousands of people are on warfarin in the UK. For safety reasons, patients must always carry a warfarin card with them in case of a medical emergency. This will tell any doctor or nurse that the person is on warfarin if there is a need for urgent treatment. Overall, it is clear that a decision to use warfarin is not straightforward and will require careful consideration by the GP or hospital specialist. As a result of these problems newer anticoagulants have been developed and are likely to be increasingly used. These include drugs such as dabigatran, rivaroxaban and apixaban.

Recent research
Cholesterol lowering with medication
Despite following a healthy, low-fat diet after a stroke, recent research has shown that taking a cholesterol-lowering tablet in addition to dietary change can help prevent strokes and heart attacks. The 'Heart Protection Study' enrolled over 20,000 British people at risk of heart attacks and strokes, and found that a moderate dose of a cholesterol-lowering tablet from the 'statin' class helped reduce premature cardiac deaths and strokes. The surprising aspect of this study was that the treatment was effective even if the patient's blood cholesterol level was considered 'normal'.

Most British people who have a stroke have a cholesterol level above the threshold used in the study (3.5 millimoles per litre) and are therefore potentially eligible for this treatment. An interesting fact to ponder is that most people in the UK have a blood cholesterol level that, if lowered, would reduce their risk of heart attacks and strokes. The public health message is clear. Current British diets are not good for the heart and brain, and measures to reduce fat in the diet will help reduce heart attacks and strokes. For the stroke survivor, lowering blood cholesterol with drugs is a new stroke prevention strategy and, furthermore, the latest research suggests that there is no upper age limit for this type of treatment.

The underlying message from this trial was that most British people with strokes have a blood cholesterol level that is an important cause of future heart attacks and strokes. A more recent trial has confirmed the benefits of cholesterol reduction for people after stroke but has also suggested that care must be taken not to use this treatment if the stroke was caused by a bleed.

Blood pressure lowering with medication

Despite following a healthy, low-salt diet after a stroke, recent research has shown that taking blood pressure-lowering tablets can help prevent strokes and heart attacks. The PROGRESS trial enrolled over 6,000 people worldwide who had had a stroke or TIA and found that moderate blood pressure-lowering tablets (in this case well-established blood pressure medication called perindopril/Coversyl or indapamide/Natrilix) helped reduce premature cardiac deaths and strokes. The surprising aspect of this study was that the treatment was effective even if the patient's blood pressure was considered 'normal'.

Most British people who have had a stroke are therefore potentially eligible for this treatment. For the stroke survivor, lowering blood pressure with drugs is a new stroke prevention strategy and, furthermore, the latest research suggests that there is no upper age limit for this type of treatment.

The underlying message from this trial was that most British people with strokes have a blood pressure level that is an important cause of future strokes and heart attacks.

More pills for secondary prevention

One consequence of this new research is that many more stroke survivors will be eligible for different pills to reduce the risk of stroke. For example, patients surviving an ischaemic stroke (a stroke caused by a blood clot) are likely to benefit from a blood-thinning tablets such as aspirin and dipyridamole, a cholesterol-lowering tablet (such as a statin), and maybe two or even three blood pressure tablets.

The prospect of taking five or six once-a-day tablets may be daunting to many people and this potential problem should be mentioned if patients are worried about the number of pills. Most people in the trials were taking a similar mix of tablets so the combination is, in general, safe and well tolerated. If taken regularly the combination of pills may more than halve the future risk of stroke, so the benefits are substantial and likely to outweigh the personal nuisance of taking regular daily medication over many years. Work is currently under way to identify whether a 'polypill' containing these common combinations of tablets can be an effective alternative to a large number of separate tablets.

Public health strategy for cholesterol and blood pressure lowering for the population

The similarities of the results of the recent cholesterol- and blood pressure-lowering trials deserve some additional comment. Both studies (discussed above) were not simply a good idea tested in a large trial. Experienced teams of researchers who had meticulously studied the patterns of heart attacks and strokes in different communities – the science of epidemiology – designed both trials. They had noticed that there wasn't a magic threshold of blood pressure or cholesterol that suddenly made you at risk of heart attacks or strokes.

In fact the evidence strongly suggested that the higher the blood pressure (and the higher the cholesterol), the higher your risk of heart attack or stroke over a large range of usual blood pressure and cholesterol ranges. In fact, these ranges include a large proportion of the healthy middle-aged and elderly British population. The trials have conclusively shown that, if you've already had a stroke, you should be considered for tablets to reduce your blood pressure and cholesterol, because you have a much higher risk of having another vascular event (such as a heart attack or stroke) than a similarly aged person who has never had a stroke.

But do the rest of us need tablets to lower our cholesterol and blood pressure? Maybe not all of us! However, the recent research sends an important public health message. Increasing blood pressure and cholesterol are a very important cause of stroke in western societies and we need to improve our lifestyles. Measures to reduce blood pressure include encouraging lifelong exercise (for example, enjoyable sports activities at schools) and stopping smoking.

The changes in legislation to stop smoking in bars and pubs in the UK have had a substantial benefit in reducing vascular events such as heart attacks and strokes due to the public health benefit of many millions of people reducing or stopping their smoking, and by eliminating secondary smoking in such venues. Dietary changes are the best way to reduce blood cholesterol and promoting lifelong daily consumption of fresh fruit and vegetables will help keep the population healthier.

Doppler scanning

Carotid Doppler scanning uses ultrasound (inaudible sound beams) to look at the flow of blood through blood vessels in the neck.

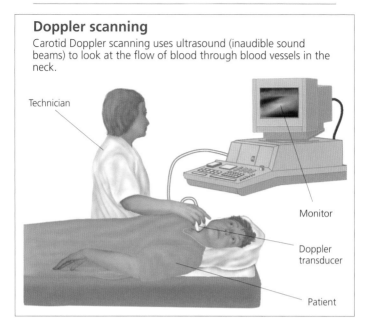

Technician

Monitor

Doppler transducer

Patient

Surgery

In some people, the stroke (or TIA) has been caused by a very tight narrowing of the carotid artery, one of the two large blood vessels in the front of the neck supplying blood to the brain. For some, an operation to clear this blockage can be worthwhile, and will help prevent future major strokes. This operation is called a carotid endarterectomy. As the operation also carries a risk of a stroke, surgery is recommended only for those people who seem to have a high chance of getting a stroke in the next few years.

Doctors use careful assessment and some special tests, such as a carotid Doppler, duplex scanning and angiography, to determine whether an operation could be worthwhile. Generally, surgery is suitable in people whose risk of having a stroke is over 20 to 30 per cent

Cerebral angiography

In cerebral angiography, a dye is injected via a catheter into an artery in the neck. The outline of the blood flow through the blood vessels is then recorded on an X-ray.

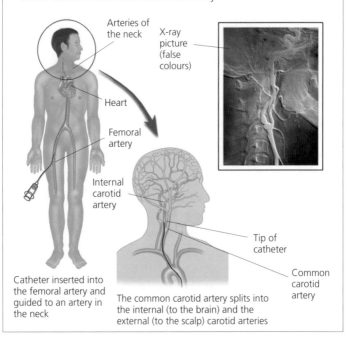

Arteries of the neck

X-ray picture (false colours)

Heart

Femoral artery

Internal carotid artery

Tip of catheter

Common carotid artery

Catheter inserted into the femoral artery and guided to an artery in the neck

The common carotid artery splits into the internal (to the brain) and the external (to the scalp) carotid arteries

in the next 2 years, that is, a 1 in 3 to 1 in 5 chance of trouble. It is important to check that the person's stroke (or TIA) was in the same part of the brain supplied by the carotid artery. The assessment should be done by groups of experts in stroke assessment, brain imaging specialists and carotid surgeons. Although the carotid blood vessel narrowing can also be treated by angioplasty (use of special catheter and balloon – see 'Glossary', page 100) and stenting (use of wire cage to open artery – see 'Glossary', page 105), recent research has confirmed that surgery is still the best option for many. However, some people may prefer to have the non-surgical method.

KEY POINTS

- Some people worry about getting back to normal activities after a stroke, but in general people should be encouraged to try to lead a normal life with no major restrictions

- People holding driving licences must let the DVLA know that they've had a stroke or TIA

- If people recover well from a stroke, they will usually be allowed to resume driving, but occupational drivers are subject to different rules

- Once someone has had a stroke, he or she is at a higher than average risk of another stroke in the future

- There are many ways to prevent a second stroke

Caring for someone after a stroke

A stroke not only affects the patient but can have a devastating effect on the family and carers. It is distressing to see a loved one affected by a stroke and relatives will have many questions and concerns. It is important that the person voices worries to the stroke team at an early stage. If matters are getting complicated with, for example, arranging a major package of care after discharge from the hospital, meetings with the family and the entire stroke team can be useful.

The move from hospital to home can appear quite daunting, especially if major adaptations of the home are required. The thought of having complete strangers in the home on a daily basis can also be upsetting, but getting outside help may be the only way for someone to return to living back home.

As stroke disease covers a wide range of problems, it is impossible to give detailed advice in a book such as this. If your relative has been affected by a stroke, you should get information from the professionals caring for him or her. The major stroke charities also provide telephone and written information (see 'Useful addresses', page 107).

Providing support

People who have just had a stroke need lots of support, not only from the stroke team but also from their family. A stroke comes on quickly but tends to improve slowly, and great patience is needed because, for some, recovery can be very slow. People need time to adjust to their new situation and this can be very stressful for family members.

If you are the main carer, it is important to establish a daily routine. The person recovering from the stroke may be more able at certain times of the day, so it is important to use this time for things that he or she most wants to do. You should also encourage the person to see friends or go out, because this will help him or her to return to normal activities.

It is important that carers are not overprotective, however, because there is a fine line between helping someone and encouraging independence. Caring for someone after a stroke can be time-consuming and frustrating, but it is important to help the person relearn skills and regain confidence, rather than do everything for him or her. It is also important to be patient, as some people will find it difficult to relearn simple tasks.

Your new role

After a relative has experienced a stroke, you may find yourself taking over new tasks or responsibilities, such as cooking or managing the family finances. This will change your daily routine and put more pressure on you. Some carers drink and smoke more, as a way of dealing with their new role, but this is not a long-term solution.

Caring for someone after a stroke can be a physical challenge. You need to learn how to lift and move someone without causing him or her or yourself an injury. You may also need to help him or her with feeding or speech difficulties. You should work with the stroke team, especially the physiotherapist and occupational therapist, to ensure that you are looking after the patient correctly. It is important that you look after yourself too. Common problems among carers include back strain, stress and fatigue.

Help for carers

Carers need support from other carers and local groups. Many areas now hold support clubs for carers and relatives, often run by charities, such as the Stroke Association or Chest, Heart & Stroke Scotland (see 'Useful addresses', pages 109 and 117). These groups can be a source of information, support and practical advice. The stroke unit may also hold meetings for relatives and carers. Support is also available through GPs, district nurses and local community rehabilitation services.

It is important that carers take regular breaks. Ask the stroke team about 'respite care', which involves care in your own home, outside your home (at day care centres, for example) or longer breaks in a nursing or residential home.

KEY POINTS

■ Caring for someone after a stroke is physically and emotionally challenging

■ Charities offer a great deal of support for relatives and carers of people who have had a stroke

Glossary

amaurosis fugax (transient monocular blindness):
a sudden blindness, often like a black shutter coming
down, affecting one eye. This is usually the result of
problems with the circulation to the brain and eye and
is a sort of mini-stroke affecting the eye. Needs to be
assessed by your doctor

aneurysm: an abnormal weak area of blood vessel wall
prone to bursting (a common cause of a subarachnoid
haemorrhage)

angioplasty: the use of a special catheter, inserted into
the artery in the leg, and passed to the blood vessels
in the neck to open up blocked arteries with a balloon.
Commonly combined with stenting (see later)

apoplexy: a very old term for stroke

artery: a blood vessel usually carrying blood pumped
from the heart to parts of the body. This is the higher
pressure part of the blood supply system

aspirin: a well-known drug that thins the blood and
prevents clotting. Used to treat patients with stroke

atherosclerosis: the medical condition that leads to the furring up and blockage of blood vessels. This damage to the blood vessels is often a source of blood clots, leading to strokes and heart attacks

atherothrombosis: the condition of abnormal blood clots forming on damaged blood vessels (atherosclerosis)

atrial fibrillation (AF): an abnormal heart condition where the heart beats irregularly, often causing palpitations; it can lead to strokes caused by abnormal blood clots formed in the heart

carotid arteries: the two main blood vessels in the front of the neck which make up two of the four main blood vessels supplying the brain

cerebrovascular accident (CVA): an old term for stroke

cerebral hemisphere: the main right and left parts of the brain are called the cerebral hemispheres. The left hemisphere usually controls the right side of the body and the right hemisphere usually controls the left side of the body. Language is controlled by the left hemisphere in right-handed people and also in about 50 per cent of left-handed people

clopidogrel: a blood-thinning agent that can help prevent stroke

CT (computed tomography) scanner: the X-ray machine that can produce detailed pictures of the body. A brain CT scan can show the cause of stroke and exclude abnormal bleeding in the brain

diabetes: a common condition that causes abnormally high levels of sugar in the body. Often needs treatment by diet, special medication or insulin

dipyridamole: a blood-thinning agent that can help prevent stroke, especially in combination with aspirin

dissection: an abnormal tear in the blood vessel wall that can cause strokes, especially if the blood vessel has been damaged by a sudden bang or pressure over the blood vessel. This can be a cause of a stroke after attempted strangulation or a sports injury

dysarthria: a problem of producing the sounds of speech. This may merely be a slurring of speech but in severe cases can mean a total loss of speech (anarthria)

dysphasia: a problem of language production. Mild forms can cause word-finding difficulties, moderate dysphasia causes muddled words and phrases, and severe cases result in no language at all (aphasia). The term is also used for difficulty in understanding speech

echocardiography: a detailed scan of the heart using ultrasound. A special probe is placed on the chest wall and the sound waves can be analysed to form pictures of the heart beating

electrocardiogram (ECG): a recording of the electrical activity of the heart by attaching wires on the arms, chest wall and legs. A very common test after a stroke as heart disease is common in people with stroke

haemorrhage: an escape of blood (abnormal bleed)

hemianopia: a loss of vision in part of the visual field. For example, some people with large strokes affecting the left side of the brain lose the ability to see to the right

hemiparesis: a weakness affecting the arm and leg on the same side of the body as a result of problems with the brain or spinal cord (often abbreviated to 'hemi' by patients and medical staff)

indapamide: a mild diuretic (water tablet) to lower blood pressure

infarct: permanent damage to body tissue (tissue death). A cerebral infarct is when part of the brain is irreversibly damaged by a blocked blood vessel

intravenous: the method of giving fluids straight into the blood supply system of the body. The veins are the low-pressure blood vessels and are relatively easy to use

ischaemic: tissue starved of a normal blood supply as a result of a blocked or narrowed blood vessel. Often leads to permanent damage, for example, a stroke in the brain

magnetic resonance imaging (MRI): a sophisticated scanning technique that uses a powerful magnet (rather than X-rays) and computer to produce detailed pictures of the body. People with metal implants (for example, an intracranial aneurysm clip or a pacemaker) cannot be scanned because the magnetic field is so powerful that it can dislodge the metal

migraine: a common medical condition characterised by flashing lights, feeling sick, a throbbing one-sided headache and an overwhelming need to lie down in a darkened room. Can be very mild or very severe. Very occasionally a severe attack can cause a stroke

occupational therapist: a therapist who helps people do everyday activities such as wash, dress, eat, make meals and use the toilet

oestrogen: a female hormone, used in the oral contraceptive pill

perindopril: a commonly used blood pressure-lowering tablet, which is also used to treat heart failure

physiotherapist: a therapist who uses movement and exercises to help people recover from stroke and other disabling conditions

primary intracerebral haemorrhage: an abnormal collection of blood in the brain resulting from a burst blood vessel (artery). The second most common cause of stroke

progestogen: a female hormone, used in the oral contraceptive pill

pulmonary embolism: a blood clot which travels to the lung and damages part of it. This can be a complication of stroke, especially if there has been a leg thrombosis. Potentially very serious and can result in death

randomised: the method of allocating clinical trial treatments in medical research. This makes sure that the doctor and patient do not cheat and choose the treatment themselves

seizure: an electrical storm in the brain often causing loss of consciousness, abnormal muscle twitching, abnormal behaviour and a short period of excessive sleepiness (or varying combinations of the above). Epilepsy is the term given to a condition with frequent attacks. A single attack can occur with the onset of stroke and stroke is the most common cause of epilepsy in older people

simvastatin: a tablet from the 'statin' group of cholesterol-lowering pills used to treat patients with heart attacks and strokes

social worker: a member of the stroke team with expertise in financial matters (for example, benefits), local services to care for patients after hospital discharge (for example, home care and meals on wheels), and assessing whether people need continuing care in residential or nursing homes. In the UK, social workers are usually employed by the local council, although they are often based within the NHS hospital

speech and language therapist: a member of the stroke team with special expertise in assessing communication and language. They have also developed a very important role in assessing the safety of the swallow mechanism and help to advise the nursing team on the best feeding methods for patients with stroke

statins: a class of cholesterol-lowering pills, which will be increasingly used to treat patients with stroke

stenting: when a blood vessel is opened up and reinforced with a wire cage to keep the blood vessel open (now used after successful angioplasty – see earlier)

stroke: a sudden onset of loss of neurological function (for example, weakness affecting arm and leg, speech problem), with symptoms that last more than 24 hours, or show up on brain scanning, resulting from a problem with the blood supply to the brain.

subcutaneous: the method of giving fluids into the body by allowing the body to absorb the fluid from under the skin. A really useful way of giving people extra fluids with few side effects

thrombolytic therapy: powerful blood clot-dissolving treatment. The main treatment for heart attacks and a promising treatment for some strokes. Unfortunately, it can cause severe bleeding in some people and more research will be needed to check that this type of treatment should be used. Recombinant tissue plasminogen activator (rtPA) and streptokinase are the most commonly used thrombolytic agents in the UK

ticlopidine: a blood-thinning agent that can prevent stroke. It is only rarely used in the UK because of important side effects on the blood. Needs to be carefully monitored with frequent blood tests

transient ischaemic attack (TIA): a mini-stroke with symptoms that fully recover in less than 24 hours (often recover within seconds or minutes). Can be a warning that a more severe stroke is about to happen. Should be assessed by a doctor

transient monocular blindness: *see* amaurosis fugax

transoesophageal echocardiography (TOE): a special heart scan by using sound waves from a tube placed in the oesophagus (gullet). Needs a skilled person to put the tube in the correct place and the patient usually requires a mild sedative or throat spray

warfarin: a commonly used tablet to thin the blood. Very useful for preventing strokes but can cause abnormal bleeding

Useful addresses

We have included the following organisations because, on preliminary investigation, they may be of use to the reader. However, we do not have first-hand experience of each organisation and so cannot guarantee the organisation's integrity. The reader must therefore exercise his or her own discretion and judgement when making further enquiries.

Abilitynet
Acre House, 11–15 William Road
London NW1 3ER
Tel: 01926 312847
Helpline: 0800 269 545
Website: www.abilitynet.org.uk

Offers advice and support on benefits of computers available to disabled children and adults. Can arrange assessment at home or at work for a fee.

Afasic

20 Bowling Green Lane
London EC1R 0BD
Tel: 020 7490 9410
Helpline: 0845 355 5577 (Mon–Fri 10.30am–2.30pm)
Website: www.afasicengland.org.uk

Offers help for people who have speech impairments.

Age UK

Tavis House, 1–6 Tavistock Square
London WC1H 9NA
Tel: 020 8765 7200
Helpline: 0800 169 6565
Website: www.ageuk.org.uk

Researches into the needs of older people and is
involved in policy-making. Publishes many books
and has useful fact sheets on a wide range of issues
from benefits to care, and provides services via local
branches.

Benefits Enquiry Line

Helpline: 0800 882200
Minicom: 0800 243355
Website: www.dwp.gov.uk
N. Ireland: 0800 220674

Government agency giving information and advice
on sickness and disability benefits for people with
disabilities and their carers.

Blood Pressure Association
60 Cranmer Terrace
London SW17 0QS
Information line 0845 241 0989 (Mon–Fri 11am–3pm)
Tel: 020 8772 4994
Website: www.bpassoc.org.uk

Raises public awareness about, and offers information
and support to, health-care professionals and people
affected by high blood pressure. Has a wide selection
of literature and membership scheme. A4 envelope and
two first-class stamps requested.

Chest, Heart & Stroke Scotland
Head Office, Third Floor, Rosebery House,
9 Haymarket Terrace, Edinburgh EH12 5EZ
Tel: 0131 225 6963
Advice line: 0845 077 6000
Website: www.chss.org.uk

Funds research, provides care and support throughout
Scotland, and has an advice line to professional advice
from trained nurse. Booklets, factsheets, DVDs and
videos available free to patients and carers.

Clinical Knowledge Summaries
Sowerby Centre for Health Informatics at Newcastle
(SCHIN Ltd), Clayton House, Clayton Road, Jesmond
Newcastle upon Tyne NE2 1TL
Tel: 0845 113 1000
Website: www.schin.co.uk

A website mainly for GPs giving information for patients
listed by disease plus named self-help organisations.

Connect – the communication disability network
16–18 Marshalsea Road
London SE1 1HL
Tel: 020 7367 0840
Website: www.ukconnect.org

Charity for people living with aphasia, a communication disability that usually occurs after a stroke.

Contact-a-Family
209–211 City Road
London EC1V 1JN
Tel: 020 7608 8700
Textphone: 0808 808 3556
Helpline: 0808 808 3555
Website: www.cafamily.org.uk

Has information on over 1,000 rare disorders and disabilities and can put families in touch with each other for mutual support.

Counsel and Care
Twyman House, 16 Bonny Street
London NW1 9PG
Tel: 020 7241 8555
Helpline: 0845 300 7585 (Mon–Fri 10am–4pm)
Website: www.counselandcare.org.uk

Offers information to people aged over 60 on welfare rights, benefits, community care. Helps with choice of residential homes, including inspection and registration of units. Some grants available.

Depression Alliance
20 Great Dover Street
London SE1 4LX
Helpline: 0845 123 2320
Website: www.depressionalliance.org

Offers support and understanding to anyone affected
by depression and for relatives who want to help. Has a
network of self-help groups, correspondence schemes and
a range of literature. An s.a.e. requested for information.

Different Strokes
9 Canon Harnett Court, Wolverton Mill
Milton Keynes MK12 5NF
Helpline: 0845 130 7172
Website: www.differentstrokes.co.uk

Stroke survivors offer information and support to
younger people who have had a stroke.

Disabled Living Foundation
380–384 Harrow Road
London W9 2HU
Tel: 020 7289 6111
Helpline: 0845 130 9177 (Mon–Fri 10am–4pm)
Textphone: 020 7432 8009
Website: www.dlf.org.uk

Provides information to disabled and elderly people
on all kinds of equipment in order to promote their
independence and quality of life.

DVLA
Driver and Vehicle Licensing Agency
Swansea SA6 7JL
Tel: 0300 790 6806
Website: www.dvla.gov.uk

Provides information about medical conditions, driving
licences, learning to drive, entitlement to drive,
endorsements/disqualifications, driving abroad and what
to do when you have changed your address and/or name.

Elderly Accommodation Counsel
Third Floor, 89 Albert Embankment
London SE1 7TP
Tel: 020 7820 1343
Website: www.eac.org.uk

Information and advice on all forms of accommodation
for elderly people, including listings of registered
nursing and care homes and sheltered housing to rent
or buy plus Social Services provision.

HemiHelp
6 Market Road
London N7 9PW
Tel: 0845 120 3713
Helpline: 0845 123 2372 (Mon–Fri 10am–1pm)
Website: www.hemihelp.org.uk

Provides information and support for children with
hemiplegia and their families. Has conferences for
medical and educational professionals to increase
public awareness of hemiplegia and its associated
conditions. Arranges fun days for children.

Institute of Child Health
30 Guilford Street
London WC1N 1EH
Website: www.ich.ucl.ac.uk

Pursues integrated multidisciplinary approach to enhance understanding, diagnosis, therapy and prevention of childhood disease, including stroke.

mobilise
National Headquarters:
Ashwellthorpe, Norwich NR16 1EX
Tel: 01508 489449
Website: www.mobilise.info

Offers information service to disabled drivers about ferries, airports and insurance. Subscription for monthly magazine.

National Institute of Conductive Education
Website: www.conductive-education.org.uk

Promotes the methods of treatment initiated by the Peto Institute, Hungary, to help children and adults affected by motor disorders. Offers training courses for professionals and families of those affected by such disorders.

National Institute for Health and Clinical Excellence (NICE)
MidCity Place, 71 High Holborn
London WC1V 6NA
Tel: 0845 003 7780
Website: www.nice.org.uk

Provides national guidance on the promotion of good health and the prevention and treatment of ill-health. Patient information leaflets are available for each piece of guidance issued.

NHS Direct
Tel: 0845 4647 (24 hours, 365 days a year)
Website: www.nhsdirect.nhs.uk

Offers confidential health-care advice, information and referral service. A good first port of call for any health advice.

NHS Smoking Helpline
Freephone: 0800 022 4332 (Mon–Fri 9am–8pm, Sat & Sun 11am–5pm)
Website: http://smokefree.nhs.uk
Pregnancy smoking helpline: 0800 169 9169 (times as above)

Have advice, help and encouragement on giving up smoking. Specialist advisers available to offer ongoing support to those who genuinely are trying to give up smoking. Can refer to local branches.

Northern Ireland Chest Heart and Stroke
21 Dublin Road
Belfast BT2 7HB
Tel: 028 9032 0184
Helpline: 0845 769 7299
Website: www.nichsa.com

Aims to promote the prevention of, and alleviate the suffering caused by chest, heart and stroke illnesses in Northern Ireland through advice and information.

Patients' Association
PO Box 935, Harrow, Middlesex HA1 3YJ
Helpline: 0845 608 4455
Tel: 020 8423 9111
Website: www.patients-association.com

Provides advice on patients' rights, leaflets and a directory of self-help groups.

Quit (Smoking Quitlines)
63 St Mary's Axe, London EC3A 8AA
Helpline: 0800 002200 (Mon–Fri 9am–8pm,
Sat 9.45am–6pm, Sun 10am–6pm)
Tel: 020 7469 0400
Website: www.quit.org.uk

Offers individual advice on giving up smoking in English and Asian languages. Talks to schools on smoking and pregnancy and can refer to local support groups. Runs training courses for professionals.

RADAR
12 City Forum, 250 City Road
London EC1V 8AF
Tel: 020 7250 3222
Minicom: 020 7250 4119
Website: www.radar.org.uk

Campaigning and advisory body run by and for disabled people. Sells key to access locked public lavatories for £3.50. Offers a range of services to its members.

Royal College of Physicians of London
11 St Andrews Place, Regent's Park
London NW1 4LE
Information centre: 020 3075 1539
Tel: 020 7935 1174
Website: www.rcplondon.ac.uk

To download a copy of the National Clinical Guidelines for Stroke.

Royal National Institute for the Blind
105 Judd Street
London WC1H 9NE
Tel: 020 7388 1266
Helpline: 0303 123 9999
Website: www.rnib.org.uk

Offers a range of information and advice on lifestyle changes and employment for people facing loss of sight. Also offers local support and training in Braille. Has mail order catalogue of useful aids.

Speakability
1 Royal Street
London SE1 7LL
Tel: 020 7261 9572
Helpline: 0808 808 9572
Website: www.speakability.org.uk

Offers information and support to people with aphasia (communication difficulties after stroke or head injury) and their families. Has self-help groups and provides training for carers and health professionals.

Stroke Association
Stroke House, 240 City Road
London EC1V 2PR
Tel: 020 7566 0300
Helpline: 0303 303 3100 (Mon–Fri 9am–5pm)
Website: www.stroke.org.uk

Funds research and provides information, now specialising only in strokes. Local support groups.

War Widows' Association
c/o 199 Borough High Street
London SE1 1AA
Tel: 0845 2412 189
Website: www.warwidowsassociation.org.uk

Campaigns on behalf of war widows in the UK, not only in times of conflict but also in peacetime. Offers information and support and can refer to other organisations as appropriate.

Useful websites
BBC
www.bbc.co.uk/health
A helpful website: easy to navigate and offers lots of useful advice and information. Also contains links to other related topics.

Behind the Gray
www.behindthegray.net
Online support for those whose lives have been
affected by a subarachnoid haemorrhage or stroke.

Bodytalkonline
www.bodytalk-online.com
Series of online presentations about different medical
conditions.

Child Stroke Support Site
www.childstrokesupport.com
Set up by parents of children who have had a stroke.

Healthtalkonline
www.healthtalkonline.org
Website of the DIPEx charity.

Medinfo
www.medinfo.co.uk
Factsheets available.

Patient UK
www.patient.co.uk
Patient care website.

The internet as a source of further information

After reading this book, you may feel that you would
like further information on the subject. The internet
is of course an excellent place to look and there are
many websites with useful information about medical
disorders, related charities and support groups.

For those who do not have a computer at home some bars and cafes offer facilities for accessing the internet. These are listed in the Yellow Pages under 'Internet Bars and Cafes' and 'Internet Providers'. Your local library offers a similar facility and has staff to help you find the information that you need.

It should always be remembered, however, that the internet is unregulated and anyone is free to set up a website and add information to it. Many websites offer impartial advice and information that have been compiled and checked by qualified medical professionals. Some, on the other hand, are run by commercial organisations with the purpose of promoting their own products. Others still are run by pressure groups, some of which will provide carefully assessed and accurate information whereas others may be suggesting medications or treatments that are not supported by the medical and scientific community.

Unless you know the address of the website you want to visit – for example, www.familydoctor.co.uk – you may find the following guidelines useful when searching the internet for information.

Search engines and other searchable sites

Google (www.google.co.uk) is the most popular search engine used in the UK, followed by Yahoo! (http://uk.yahoo.com) and MSN (www.msn.co.uk). Also popular are the search engines provided by Internet Service Providers such as Tiscali and other sites such as the BBC site (www.bbc.co.uk).

In addition to the search engines that index the whole web, there are also medical sites with search facilities, which act almost like mini-search engines, but cover only medical topics or even a particular area of medicine. Again, it is wise to look at who is responsible for compiling the information offered to ensure that it is impartial and medically accurate. The NHS Direct site (www.nhsdirect.nhs.uk) is an example of a searchable medical site.

Links to many British medical charities can be found at the Association of Medical Research Charities' website (www.amrc.org.uk) and at Charity Choice (www.charitychoice.co.uk).

Search phrases

Be specific when entering a search phrase. Searching for information on 'cancer' will return results for many different types of cancer as well as on cancer in general. You may even find sites offering astrological information. More useful results will be returned by using search phrases such as 'lung cancer' and 'treatments for lung cancer'. Both Google and Yahoo! offer an advanced search option that includes the ability to search for the exact phrase; enclosing the search phrase in quotes, that is, 'treatments for lung cancer', will have the same effect. Limiting a search to an exact phrase reduces the number of results returned but it is best to refine a search to an exact match only if you are not getting useful results with a normal search. Adding 'UK' to your search term will bring up mainly British sites, so a good phrase might be 'lung cancer' UK (don't include UK within the quotes).

Always remember that the internet is international and unregulated. It holds a wealth of valuable information but individual sites may be biased, out of date or just plain wrong. Family Doctor Publications accepts no responsibility for the content of links published in this series.

Index

Your pages

We have included the following pages because they may help you manage your illness or condition and its treatment.

Before an appointment with a health professional, it can be useful to write down a short list of questions of things that you do not understand, so that you can make sure that you do not forget anything.

Some of the sections may not be relevant to your circumstances.

We are always pleased to receive constructive criticism or suggestions about how to improve the books. You can contact us at:

Email: familydoctor@btinternet.com
Letter: Family Doctor Publications
         PO Box 4664
         Poole
         BH15 1NN

Thank you

Health-care contact details

Name:

Job title:

Place of work:

Tel:

Name:

Job title:

Place of work:

Tel:

Name:

Job title:

Place of work:

Tel:

Name:

Job title:

Place of work:

Tel:

Significant past health events – illnesses/ operations/investigations/treatments

Event	Month	Year	Age (at time)

Appointments for health care

Name:

Place:

Date:

Time:

Tel:

Name:

Place:

Date:

Time:

Tel:

Name:

Place:

Date:

Time:

Tel:

Name:

Place:

Date:

Time:

Tel:

Appointments for health care

Name:

Place:

Date:

Time:

Tel:

Name:

Place:

Date:

Time:

Tel:

Name:

Place:

Date:

Time:

Tel:

Name:

Place:

Date:

Time:

Tel:

Current medication(s) prescribed by your doctor

Medicine name:

Purpose:

Frequency & dose:

Start date:

End date:

Medicine name:

Purpose:

Frequency & dose:

Start date:

End date:

Medicine name:

Purpose:

Frequency & dose:

Start date:

End date:

Medicine name:

Purpose:

Frequency & dose:

Start date:

End date:

Other medicines/supplements you are taking, not prescribed by your doctor

Medicine/treatment:

Purpose:

Frequency & dose:

Start date:

End date:

Medicine/treatment:

Purpose:

Frequency & dose:

Start date:

End date:

Medicine/treatment:

Purpose:

Frequency & dose:

Start date:

End date:

Medicine/treatment:

Purpose:

Frequency & dose:

Start date:

End date:

Questions to ask at appointments
(Note: do bear in mind that doctors work under great time pressure, so long lists may not be helpful for either of you)

Questions to ask at appointments
(Note: do bear in mind that doctors work under great time pressure, so long lists may not be helpful for either of you)

Notes